THIN FOR LIFE

THIN FOR LIFE

A Program of Permanent Weight
Control as Originally Developed
at Duke University

Richard G. Stuelke, M.D.

Baronet Publishing Company, NEW YORK, 1977

International Standard Book Number: 0-89437-000-6
Library of Congress Catalog Card Number: 77-2469

Manufactured in the United States of America

First Printing

Baronet Publishing Company, New York, N.Y. 10022

Library of Congress Cataloging in Publication Data

Stuelke, Richard G   1933-
    Thin for Life

    1. Low-calorie diet—Recipes. 2. Reducing—Psychological aspects. 3. Obesity—Psychological aspects. 4. Food habits. I. Title. [DNLM: 1. Diet, Reducing. 2. Obesity—Therapy—Popular works. 3. Behavior therapy—Popular works. WD212 S933p]
RM222.2.S87   613.2'5   77-2469
ISBN 0-89437-000-6

My grateful appreciation to . . .

. . . Duke University, where I first developed and perfected my program of positive, permanent weight control;

. . . to the thousands of patients who have controlled their obesity problems through the application of the principles of psychostructure;

. . . to HARRY PRESTON, for his valuable editorial assistance in the preparation of this manuscript.

Richard G. Stuelke, M.D.

CONTENTS

INTRODUCTION

Another book on weight control? Aren't there enough already on the market? Certainly there are, and most professionally written diet books can help you lose weight *temporarily* provided you stick to the prescribed dietary guidelines; but therein lies the problem for those of us who suffer from obesity: by our very natures, we are unable to limit our food intake on a *permanent* basis.

We may be able to endure brief periods during which we stoically deny ourselves our usual massive helpings at mealtimes; but after we can smile instead of shudder when we step on a bathroom scale, we inevitably return to our former eating habits and start the battle of the bulge once again. The obvious conclusion is that permanent weight control involves more than merely going on a diet.

I know this fact only too well. In 1968, I weighed nearly 300 pounds. From my medical background as well as my growing personal discomfort, I realized that unless I found a way to lose weight permanently, I would continue to miss much that life has to offer. I might even lose my life prematurely, obesity often being directly associated with disease processes which contribute to a shorter life.

But, you may say at this point: *I* do not suffer from obesity.

I'm just a little overweight. However, that's like the young woman who said she was just a little pregnant!

Either you are or you are not over your ideal weight for your height and age. No amount of semantic side-stepping will change that fact, so let's be blunt about the problem.

Technically, obesity is defined as your ideal weight plus twenty percent. However, the problem involves considerably more than a simple definition. Therefore, in this book I shall refer more to *obesity* than to *overweight* or *fat* or other terms that you might consider more palatable. Why? Because *anyone* who tips the scale at more than his ideal weight needs to face the facts about this problem. Only by knowing the truth can we be set free from the burden of carrying excess flab on our bodies.

I know only too well the burden of which I speak, which is why, in 1968, I went to Duke University for treatment. At that time, Duke University had begun treating certain types of heart disease with a diet using rice as a mainstay. The diet had proved to be beneficial in weight reduction as well, so I entered the program.

I lost one hundred pounds. Later, regrettably I gained it all back. The rice diet, like many other programs that limit the type and amount of food we eat, is effective only when strictly adhered to, and no one wants to exist on rice for a lifetime.

Similarly, there are dozens of so-called miracle diets and drugs that may pare inches off your waistline in a few months, but the results are temporary, not permanent. Most people who go this route find themselves sliding back up the scale when they inevitably resume their former eating habits.

I decided to devote my time to discovering a permanently effective treatment for this disease—for *obesity is a disease* that affects more than forty percent of the population of the United States, as well as millions more throughout the world. In 1972, I returned to Duke University, not as a patient, but as a doctor specializing in the research and treatment of obesity.

Since my earlier visit, a low-calorie, high-protein diet had been developed by Dr. Siegfried Heyden. I found it excellent and prescribed it for patients in my Dietary Rehabilitation Clinic.

Nonetheless, the thought still nagged at my mind: diet alone was not the final answer. I had proved that myself. There had to be something more—perhaps some unknown element yet to be discovered.

Although years of painstaking effort went into my final analysis and ultimate solution to the problem of obesity, the actual turning point came to me in a flash, just as almost every major medical breakthrough has usually occurred in a most unexpected way, at an unpredictable moment—that split second when man is touched by a spark of inspiration.

One noontime I was sitting in the cafeteria at Duke University. I had just finished my lunch (150 calories!) when I suddenly realized how many of the students were overweight—young men lacking the firm, flat stomachs of high school football players, and young buxom women with soft looking, too well-rounded figures.

These overweight specimens all bustled in excitedly, approaching the steam tables with obvious anticipation, almost drooling at the display of tempting dishes. As they piled their trays high, they exchanged enthusiastic comments over the food; then they hurried to sit at the nearest table and attacked their plates as though they hadn't eaten in weeks. Yet, I suspected, they had all probably eaten a large breakfast only hours before. Then why this frantic orgy of eating?

My curiosity aroused, I turned my attention to those students who did not have an obvious weight problem. They entered the cafeteria quite briskly, would purposefully select a single dish, and move down the line with a minimum of delay. When they reached a table, they sat and consumed their lunch without the outward ecstatic delight of their plumper classmates.

Then it happened—my own flash of inspiration! I realized these two groups of students were exhibiting two totally opposite attitudes toward their food.

The overweight students gave vent to groans and gurgles of delight at the very sight of the steam table, then reached compulsively for large amounts of the most calorie-laden concoctions: lasagna, spaghetti, mashed potatoes, and fluffy cream pies.

The slender students, on the other hand, seemed to preselect what they wanted and were immune to the stimulating temptations set before them. They took one dish only (meat or fish, I noted) with one vegetable or a salad; and that was it.

Suppose, I began reasoning to myself, the plump students had the same approach toward food as their slender friends? Would they still be reaching compulsively for everything in sight, unable to be satisfied with a single, simple dish? What was causing this apparently uncontrollable urge to gorge themselves? It had to be something more than hunger. Was it perhaps their *attitudes* that were to blame? Was it some *psychological* compulsion which drove them to eat excessively?

That day in the cafeteria at Duke University proved to be the turning point in my long search for an effective treatment for obesity. For years I understandably had been concentrating my efforts on trying to arrive at the ideal food combination to prescribe for those suffering from overweight. Finally, I realized that no matter what *diets* were consumed, most people would inevitably revert to former eating habits, just as I did myself after following the rice diet. Few of us have the self discipline needed to restrict our intake of food over a prolonged period, much less permanently.

Why? The answer is simply our minds keep telling us: we're "on a diet" and once we've shed a desired number of pounds, we can thankfully go back to eating all those goodies again! A diet, therefore, assumes the nature of an *episode* of perfection and deprivation—a truly miserable period in our lives. We tend to forget that being obese is the *continuous* period of misery.

Do not believe anyone who claims to enjoy being fat! That's pure baloney—which, incidentally, is thirty-two percent fat! I have yet to meet an overweight man or woman who does not deeply crave to be slender and able to enjoy life to the fullest. So if fat people yearn to be slender, why do they continue to overeat?

The answer to this question came after an intensive and long period of research into the psychological aspects of food consumption in obese people.

I discovered a major difference between thin people and fat people: thin people refrain from overeating because of an internal control mechanism, an inherent psychological restraint that is lacking in fat people. Obese people react compulsively and spontaneously to the presence of food in their environment. This was a conclusion reinforced by my experience in the cafeteria: the thin students showed no overt reaction to the display of food; whereas the overweight students reacted immediately to the presence of food.

The validity of my conclusion was born out in experiments conducted by an eminent psychologist, Stanley J. Shackner, Ph.D., professor of psychology at Columbia University, who documented the varying responses to the presence of food in a group of thin and fat people. (Details of these experiments are given later in this book).

This phase of my research led ultimately to one of the cardinal rules in my program: it is necessary to restructure the environment of an obese person so that food is, wherever possible, completely out of reach. *Out of sight, out of mind . . .*

I discovered that obese people have no idea how much food they consume each day. Even when "on a diet" they believe they have ingested only 1500 calories, when in reality, the figure may be closer to 5000! This realization told me that some form of daily record would be essential for an obese person to be aware of his daily intake of food, down to the last calorie—because *every calorie counts!*

Faithfully and honestly keeping a daily diary is an essential part of my program, not only as a physical record of food consumed, but also as a psychological reinforcement for the individual to watch what he eats, and not only structured meals but also "unstructured" eating, such as a handful of nuts at a party.

In addition to the lack of an internal control mechanism, obese people have different eating habits than thin people. While thin people ingest their food at a leisurely pace, fat people tend to wolf their meals, a significant factor in their increased consumption of food.

In the course of observations at social gatherings, I propounded my LAW OF THE COCKTAIL PARTY: *The distance between the hors d'oeuvre table and the guest is inversely proportional to his weight.*

Similarly, through personal observation and patient contact, I discovered the LAW OF THE SPECTATOR. *The straightness of the line between the box office and the candy counter is directly proportional to the customer's weight.* The Law of the Spectator primarily grew out of my experience with Bobby S., the teenage son of a man who owns a chain of theaters in a large Eastern city. Understandably, Bobby grew up attending every movie he had time for; which was almost every day and most nights.

By the time Bobby was seventeen, he had a serious weight problem. He came to me for treatment, and began doing very well on the diet I prescribed; he claimed he was eating only those items I specified for each meal.

Nevertheless, his weight loss was minimal. It was then I learned that his lifestyle included daily attendance at one of his father's many theaters. Did he eat anything while at a movie? Of course! Popcorn, ice cream, soft drinks. Why not? He didn't have to pay for it. But, I pointed out, you are paying for it with those extra unwanted pounds that are bulging around your waistline. Bobby S. eventually received the message loud and clear, particularly when I insisted that he continue to attend the theater but only to watch the movie; he could *not* eat a single morsel during the performance. Then he began making excellent progress. Eventually he achieved his desired ideal weight level, and today when he goes to see a show, he never goes near the popcorn stand. He has successfully accomplished, and is to be complimented for, his self-structuring. Patience, perseverance and self-structuring are prerequisites to success in losing weight. After all, self-structuring is better than self-destructing, which is what that time-bomb of fat can do, especially with middle-aged people with heart trouble.

While my research pointed to obese people being innately *reactive* to food, I also found they are not *active* individuals. They are essentially sedentary and do not move about or indulge in exercise the way a thin person normally does. A thin person will think nothing of walking two blocks to the store; a fat person will instinctively get in the car and drive the distance. This revelation underlined the crucial necessity for daily exercise as a major part of a successful weight-loss program, as well as restructuring the environment and, most important of all, restructuring a person's outlook and attitudes toward food; in brief, restructuring his very lifestyle.

A "diet" will always be essential to the reduction of body weight to a desired ideal level, but the maintenance of that desired level can only be permanently possible when there is a viable substitute present for the internal control mechanism that is lacking in the psychological makeup of every obese person.

Considering our present day lifestyle, I knew this was not going to be an easy task. From the moment we are born, food is associated not so much with satisfying hunger, but with satisfying our sensual urges. From the child who is given candy to quiet his cries to the adult who snacks at the cocktail party, almost everyone is programmed to regard eating as a pleasure rather than as a means to support life.

Obviously, to arrive at a totally workable program to control obesity, I had to concentrate on the areas of mental responses; to find a way to reprogram the minds of those who are unable to resist reaching out for food. Reprogramming is, in reality, psychological restructuring . . . PSYCHOSTRUCTURE!

A fancy word, you might say, but in the years since that moment in the cafeteria at Duke University, I have demonstrated through the success of scores of patients at my clinic that my program *works*.

What does it involve?

From the brief mentions above of how I arrived at my final solution to obesity, you might think it consists of a highly restrictive diet, removal of all food from the house, hours of back-breaking exercise, and reams of paper in your daily diary—all of which raises an immediate picture of a lifetime of frustrating self-denial and agony.

In your present frame of mind, this could be true; but, as many people will testify, after psychological restructuring, you too will experience no resistance to the regimen. Your new lifestyle (and your new, slender figure!) will make you feel your former fat self was nothing but a bad dream from which you have finally awakened.

Psychostructure is the introduction of an intellectual mechanism by which you can gain control over the ingestion of food. The program encompasses a knowledge of calories, knowing how to react to food, how to determine how much and when to eat, how to engage in the act of eating, and where the pitfalls lie and how to cope with them.

Psychostructure embraces not only ideas, but also is an effective working tool through which you will learn how to restructure your lifestyle and eating habits in order to achieve a desired weight loss and, thereafter, to maintain a normal healthy body weight as long as you live.

That's what this book is all about—a demonstrably effective system of losing weight permanently and staying slim for the rest of your life.

As a first and very important step toward psychostructure memorize these four basic cardinal rules:

ONE: OUT OF SIGHT, OUT OF MIND . . . restructure your environment away from the temptation of food.

TWO: EVERY CALORIE COUNTS . . . keep an accurate and honest diary of everything you eat every day.

THREE: EAT SLOWLY, TAKE YOUR TIME . . . remember the *faster* you eat the *more* you will eat.

FOUR: BE PATIENT, PERSEVERE . . . you're changing your way of life and learning a way to be permanently free of flab; don't be easily discouraged and lapse into former bad habits, as self-satisfying as they may seem to be.

1. MYTHS AND MISCONCEPTIONS ABOUT DIETING

L et me stress that *psychostructure* is not something you try for a few months to lose a few pounds. This program is a completely new lifestyle involving not only a change in your eating habits, but also a basic change in your very life that will result in your reaching and maintaining your normal, natural weight, which is as it should be. Health is everyone's right as a human being, and being overweight is not only unnatural but also unhealthy.

The Bible says, "Ye Must Be Born Again"—and that is exactly what will happen to you after completing a program of psychostructure.

You *will* be born again—into a trim, healthy, and vigorous body.

It is not that you *may*, but that you *will* achieve success. My supreme confidence in psychostructure stems from scores of individuals who have proved that this system works . . . men and women who have waddled into my clinic, panting, puffy, and pessimistic, and who have been transformed into bright, optimistic, and active people whose minds are alert and whose bodies are slender and bubbling with energy.

One vital point, however, must be stressed: *you* have to do your part, for in the final analysis, *you* are the only person who can bring about your transformation. *Your* success will be in direct proportion to your determination to follow every step of the program. You will need to understand the principles of psychostructure, and you will need perseverance and patience in following this program.

Psychostructure is not popping a pill or merely cutting down on certain foods, as some weight-control programs prescribe. You have to adopt a completely new attitude towards the problem of obesity, which is why I stress the importance of the mind, for *attitudes are mental.* You will be transformed by the renewing of your mind, and therein lies the key to making a success of psychostructure.

Most people do not realize the limitless potential of the mind. We are, after all, limited only by our imaginations and by the degree to which we utilize our mental capacities.

Unfortunately (but understandably) mankind has, over the centuries, been conditioned to believe that unless you can touch it, feel it, or see it it cannot exist. Yet everything we know began as an idea in someone's mind, from the unknown individual who invented the wheel up to such giants as Marconi, Edison, and Jonas Salk and, we all pray, for the emergence of that divinely inspired researcher of the future from whose mind will spring the cure for cancer. Do not ever sell the mind short: it is the key to all our accomplishments.

Only recently the academic fraternity has begun delving into the mysteries of mental power. Some major universities now have departments of parapsychology, investigating supernatural and super-normal phenomena, and individuals who have cultivated their mental powers to an extraordinary degree.

It would be foolish to say everyone will be able to lop off those extra pounds merely by willing the body to lose weight; but you can very effectively condition your mind to control your actions automatically, change your lifestyle, and adopt a pattern of food consumption and physical activity that results in a permanently healthy body with a normal weight.

But before you can effect a permanent change in your body, you have to effect a permanent change in your mind by clearing out all those preconceived ideas about weight control and by understanding the principles of psychostructure.

You may have the idea, conscious or subconscious, that nothing can be done about your obesity. You may believe that unless you take some form of medication to "melt away the fat," you will never reduce. You may think that strenuous prolonged exercises are mandatory, or that you must give up all your favorite foods. There are dozens of false ideas that have arisen to make the idea of permanent weight control an impossible dream for many people. I know. I have listened to hundreds of sad stories over the past few years, all of which reinforced my contention that too many people stay fat because they believe this is their lot in life. They have unconsciously brainwashed themselves into accepting their condition as hopeless. No obese condition is hopeless! People on this program have lost in excess of 300 pounds! Believe me, psychostructure *works! Believe.* Beliefs are mental, and stem from prior inputs into your mind.

The first step in psychostructure is a mental housecleaning, replacing untrue and detrimental ideas about weight control with positive, factual information on which to rebuild your attitudes and restructure your outlook. To accomplish this, a proper understanding of obesity is necessary; an understanding that dispels popular myths.

Many men and women suffer from the delusion that they were born fat and there is absolutely nothing they can do about it. Not so. Certain genetic traits may be passed on from generation to generation, but plump parents do not always produce a brood of butterballs. Inherited obesity still remains only a theory, and as such is open to questioning. No matter what the cause of obesity may be, psychostructure works.

Then there are those who believe that "fat can be beautiful." I don't buy this idea at all. If fat *were* so appealing, why is it almost every fat person wants to lose weight?

In certain cultures a plump female is considered the epitome of pulchritude, but in our Western civilization a slim body is preferred, not only for aesthetic reasons, but for the more important reasons of health and longevity. Obesity not only limits your enjoyment of life, but limits your very lifespan.

That brings us to the matter of exercise, which is possibly the most misunderstood aspect of any weight control program. Many people think that exercise doesn't do any good. They quote the statement that you have to walk thirty-six miles to lose one pound of fat, which happens to be true. But let's be reasonable: excess weight does not appear overnight. The buildup of fat takes weeks, months, sometimes years, and it is ridiculous to consider losing it in a few weeks. Achieving permanent weight loss is impossible in a short space of time, which is precisely why exercise cannot reduce weight except over a prolonged period of time.

Steady, sensible exercise is essential to our health, but by walking two miles a day, you will only lose about an ounce. BUT, *an ounce a day adds up to twenty-five pounds in a year!* Many people troubled with obesity today could be enjoying a normal weight if, in addition to their present activity, they had walked two miles a day over the last two years, which would account for fifty pounds potential weight loss irrespective of the amount or type of food consumed.

Exercise means just that: physical effort, not short cuts at the health club! Machines, vibrator belts, rollers and the like, as well as massage, are absolutely useless as an effective, permanent method of weight control. The only person benefiting from massage is the masseur! And the only person benefiting from the machines is the local electric company! A steam bath is equally ineffectual; you lose only water and not body weight. The only exercise at a health club which benefits you is physical exertion brought about by your own efforts, contracting and toning the muscles and tissue.

I must interject a word of warning about steam baths: if you take a steam bath or a sauna while on a diet, especially a salt-free diet, there is the possibility of contraction of your blood supply. You have probably noticed in the past how red your skin will get in a steam room. This is caused by the concentration of blood under the skin. If you stand up quickly, there can be insufficient blood flowing to the brain, causing blacking out, or worse, a stroke. Instead of making you feel good, a steam bath or sauna can often have very damaging results, especially if you are over forty when the circulatory system is less responsive.

A major fallacy about exercise and weight control concerns exercising after a meal, which is generally regarded as inadvisable. After a meal, the body temperature rises. This is called a thermal response and results from the actual burning of calories to digest the food. Exercise causes a rise in the thermal response, and it prolongs the process, resulting in a greater consumption of calories. Walking immediately after a meal will burn off about eighteen percent more calories than if you walk before the meal. So exercising after a meal is highly recommended as an important part of a weight-control program.

Most smokers believe they will automatically gain weight if they quit smoking. This may be true unless a very structured diet is adopted to counteract the change in metabolic rate and the tendency to overeat which occur after a person stops smoking. Since psychostructure includes a controlled diet, it is possible to quit smoking during the program and not be concerned about adversely affecting your weight loss.

Yet another myth concerning weight loss involves the use of special diet drinks and diet foods. Many people have told me they felt they had to give up what they called "normal food" in order to lose weight. Nothing could be farther from the truth. I recommend only easily obtainable "normal" foods, which do not include the frequently advertised short-cut diet foods that promise "a complete meal in a glass" or some other nonsense. Products of this sort are virtually worthless in any continuing program for permanent weight control simply because you cannot exist on them forever.

The primary reason that such food products are ineffective involves what is referred to as "the satiety response"—the psychological satisfaction you get when you consume a meal.

A sense of satisfaction is absent after swallowing a glass of "instant breakfast" because you miss the seeing, smelling, chewing, and swallowing of solid food which are all integral parts of the physical and psychological ingredients of a meal.

Merely ingesting a glassful of food substitute leaves you still feeling hungry, and with a painful sense of self-denial which makes dieting an almost impossible chore. With psychostructure, you will feel none of this sense of deprivation because you will be psychologically conditioned to be satisfied even though in reality you will probably have eaten less than your usual intake.

The biggest myth of all is that in order to lose weight, you need not give up anything at all; you merely have to cut down on quantity. WRONG. There *will* be certain foods that you have to eliminate completely from your diet—but, and *this is the secret to psychostructure,* through your psychological restructuring, you will experience very little feeling of denial and frustration. It will not seem like a hardship. After eating you will feel that you have had a good meal, and there will also be the immeasurable satisfaction of knowing that what you have eaten will not add to your obesity, but is a step towards eliminating it *permanently.*

There are three basic physical types among humans and an ability to be able to identify each type will have a bearing upon your understanding of obesity and how it may be cured.

The first type is the *ectomorph,* or test tube as it is sometimes called: long boned and slender or tall and thin. Ectomorphs seldom, if ever, suffer from obesity. They eat less than other types, and their weight seems to remain constant throughout their lifetime.

The second type, the *mesomorph,* or wine glass, is the classic athletic type with broad shoulders and narrow hips. Mr. America himself. Mesomorphs look terrific at twenty, but unless they're careful, they can bloat into mountains of flab at forty.

And third, there is the *endomorph,* who is tubby and pear-shaped, with narrow shoulders, wide hips, and little muscle. Of the three basic types, the third, the endomorph, is most prone to obesity, and I have found that many endomorphs believe they have only to lose weight and they will be transformed into a Mr. America. Not so.

No weight-loss program, psychostructure included, can alter your basic physical type. Just as you have to be honest in your efforts in psychostructure, so also must you be honest about what you basically *are.* The endomorph will never look the same as a mesomorph, but whatever your type, being slim certainly gives you a better shape than being fat! I mention this to avoid any possible disappointment you may feel if, after achieving your normal weight, you don't suddenly look like Steve Reeves or Raquel Welch!

Just as there are myths about obesity itself, there are a number of misconceptions about the physical process of weight loss. Everyone who has ever gone on a diet has usually started off filled with enthusiasm and determination. They anticipate that within a few weeks, they will have dropped twenty pounds and be well on the way to achieving the figure they desire. Despite elaborate advertising claims, this just doesn't happen! Losing weight and regaining a permanently slender body takes time. The heavier you are, the longer it takes, which is why I stress patience, perseverance, and strict adherence to the total program.

The vast amount of misleading information disseminated about weight control has resulted in many people taking a diet into their own hands. Dieting is not a do-it-yourself project.

One of the greatest fallacies is that many people who go on a diet believe their rate of weight loss can be greatly increased by reducing their calorie intake below the recommended level in their diet.

This is not only untrue, but is something to be avoided because it can be harmful to your health. Suppose you were to reduce your daily caloric intake from 700 to 500. If you were able to stick to such a strict limitation for one month, your weight loss would be only a pound and a half more. In other words, 200 calories *less* per day for thirty days would only lop a pound and a half off your weight compared with what you would lose if you were getting 700 calories a day. This very minor additional weight loss presupposes that with this marked caloric restriction, your metabolism will remain the same. This is not necessarily true.

Cutting calories to 700 a day will cause some decrease in your metabolic rate; but below 700, another mechanism takes over—the same process that occurs during actual starvation, which is the body's way of staying alive. Calories are burned at a much slower rate, thereby getting the maximum possible benefit out of every bite of food. For someone lost at sea, with minimal rations to sustain life, this automatic bodily function can mean the difference between survival and starving to death; but for the overly eager dieter, this process doesn't help at all!

You know you are on a diet, which is why you are stoically suffering through a drastically reduced food intake, but your *body* doesn't know this. It reacts as though, for whatever reason, you are approaching starvation level, and performs accordingly. As a result, your weight loss will be slowed. Dropping your calories below 700 a day actually can be counter-productive to your efforts to lose weight.

There is no denying you *will* lose a little more weight at first on 500 calories a day—but the loss will not be all fat. It will be water space, because the amount of sodium in 500 calories of food is naturally less than 700 calories. When the sodium content in your diet is reduced, the water space drops accordingly, and you are not interested in losing water space.

If your caloric intake is too low, you will also find your pulse rate falling, which reduces your rate of energy burn. Your desire to exercise diminishes. And since it doesn't take too much exercise to burn off 200 calories, you're really not gaining anything by decreasing your diet below 700 calories a day.

In fact, reducing calories too low can be harmful because the body does not differentiate between protein and fat when it's burning calories. Except for a small amount of dietary fat to absorb vitamins, the major food need of the body is protein. If you fail to maintain an adequate protein level in your diet, you are liable to wind up losing protein as well as fat when you diet, because both are lost when calories are burned, and losing protein means loss of muscle mass and organ mass; the heart and the liver become smaller. All of which is a further illustration of what I said earlier: dieting is *not* a do-it-yourself project!

You must recognize another extremely important and destructive fallacy which is the idea that you can maintain a desired daily caloric level by skipping meals. Many people skip breakfast and lunch, believing that they can just as easily use up their daily ration of calories in one big meal that will be more satisfying than three smaller meals. Wrong again!

If you go all day without eating, you will be so hungry by dinner time that you are liable to gorge yourself, rationalizing your excesses by considering them a "reward" for having starved yourself. This is no mere supposition: it is a psychological fact, called the "deprivation syndrome." In other words, you feel because you have deprived yourself of breakfast and lunch, you are justified in eating a little bit more for dinner. The "little bit more" is never that; it's always *much* more.

Again, this illustrates the power of your psychostructure for in the deprivation syndrome, it's your *mental* attitude that causes your downfall, which is why restructuring your responses safeguards you against any slipping off your schedule.

The psychostructure diet divides your daily allowable calories among three meals, resulting in a continuing source of energy for your body—energy which you will need for the exercise that is also an essential part of the program. Furthermore (and most importantly), your diet must be structured in such way that after your initial weight loss, you can continue the diet to maintain your desired body weight.

In other words, you adopt a *structured* eating routine in order to lose your excess weight. During your period of weight loss, as well as afterwards, your psychological restructuring will enable you to maintain your dietary limitations and will, in time, automatically guard you against reaching out for those foods you must avoid, or becoming *unstructured,* which means losing control over what you eat and which has resulted in your becoming overweight.

One of the most curious beliefs among some dieters is the false idea that weight loss can be speeded up by inducing more frequent bowel movements through the use of laxatives. This is utterly foolish and dangerous as well. The contents of the bowel weigh very little, but it is more important to pay attention to the fact that a laxative can wash potassium out of your system, thereby depriving your body of a vital and necessary mineral.

If you adhere strictly to the psychostructure diet you will experience infrequent bowel movements, a condition called "obstipation" rather than constipation. This is not a health hazard, as *it is not necessary to have a bowel movement every day to be healthy.*

If, however, while dieting you experience not only infrequent bowel movements but also hard stools, this can indicate true constipation, in which case I suggest you check with your doctor who can advise whether or not you should use a stool softener, such as *Serutan, Metamucil,* or *Diocytal Sodium Sulfasuccinate.* One word of caution: Never combine a stool softener with mineral oil, because of the risk of possibly inducing an impaction, which does constitute a serious health problem.

Some people also believe diuretics (fluid pills) help the body lose weight. The controlled use of a diuretic can be useful, especially for women whose metabolism sometimes makes it difficult to get rid of water; but for most dieters, the practice of taking diuretics regularly, or in unprescribed large doses, is very harmful.

Diuretics deplete the system of sodium and potassium and block the excretion of uric acid. Prolonged and heavy usage can result in diabetes and gout and can increase the appetite, which is not very helpful to anyone trying to lose weight. You should only take a diuretic if it has been prescribed by your doctor. In fact, you should, as a general rule of health, only use medications of any type after consulting a doctor.

This is especially true when you are on a diet, because both your need and your tolerance for drugs can change drastically when you alter your eating habits. Check with your doctor, especially if you are taking such drugs as insulin, orinase, diuretics or hypertensive medication, as very often the drug dosage will have to be adjusted.

If you start treating yourself you are running a dangerous risk of taking a medication that may be incompatible with a drug you are already taking. When you are given a prescription for a new drug, make certain your doctor is aware of any other medication you may be taking at the time. This is especially important if you indulge yourself in appetite depressants as a presumed aid in your weight loss. Not only are these pills totally worthless for a permanently effective program of weight control, but some of them —the amphetamines—can also be extremely dangerous as they can lead to drug dependency and abuse. There may be a temporary benefit from appetite depressants, but it is short lived and will soon create a rebound effect wherein your appetite increases to a greater degree than you experienced before taking the medication.

Just as you should always check with your doctor prior to taking any type of medication, you should also consult with him before going on a diet—*any diet,* my own included.

If you were to come to my clinic, a checkup is the first step taken before prescribing a suitable diet for you. Why? Because anyone wanting to lose weight must follow a diet that is not only effective, but which will not jeopardize his health. Each one of us has our own particular set of tolerances, allergies, and reactions, both to food and to medication. Before anyone can prescribe a diet that is suitable for you, he must be certain that your overweight condition is the only problem needing attention.

Most obese people take it for granted that their only problem is being too fat, which is potentially a dangerous assumption. Hyperlipidemia, hypertension, and diabetes, to name but a few, are common conditions in an overweight person; and not all problems are necessarily related to obesity.

A pre-diet physical examination by your doctor is absolutely essential, not only to determine your present state of health, but also to discover any condition that would need attention and which might possibly be aggravated by blithely embarking on a restricted dietary program. It is also advantageous to have your doctor fully aware of what you plan to do. After all, he has been watching over your health for a number of years, presumably; he may even have attempted to help you with your weight problem in the past, probably without success, because in *any* attempt to permanently reduce weight, successful treatment depends more on the patient than the doctor.

I am confident that your doctor will welcome the news of your embarking on the psychostructure program, since it has been proven successful over the past few years at the Duke University Dietary Rehabilitation Clinic and at my own clinic as well. The system is known to be effective for those who follow it faithfully, and your doctor will doubtless rejoice at the prospect of helping you finally overcome your obesity.

In addition to a thorough physical examination, I recommend that you have a chemical profile—including urinalysis, a blood count, and a stool test for blood—done as well. An electrocardiagram should also be taken, especially for people over thirty, as well as a glucose tolerance test to check for hypoglycemia which is a rather common complaint with overweight men and women.

There are almost endless lists of bodily ailments directly and indirectly caused by obesity, and the most serious is the risk of heart attack. However, I prefer not to use scare tactics, and for a very good reason. The mere fact that you have bought this book and are reading it indicates that you plan to do something about your overweight problem. You obviously do not need further convincing that you have a serious problem with your health, and that you must do something about it now or suffer very serious consequences later.

So rather than dwell on all the negative aspects and potential health hazards of being overweight, I prefer to place my emphasis on the positive side. Accentuating the positive—as the old song goes—will serve to reinforce your determination to succeed with psychostructure even though you may have failed with other methods in the past.

It is crucial for you to remember that your success in any program of weight control lies with *you,* and if you follow the psychostructure program faithfully, stick to the prescribed diet, and work hard on restructuring your mind, *you can and will succeed* in regaining a normal healthy body weight and maintaining it for the rest for your life.

Remember the First Commandment of Psychostructure: *My success in losing weight is in direct proportion to my determination to follow every step of the program.*

2. CAUSES AND CONSEQUENCES OF OBESITY

Psychostructure is no gimmicky term dreamed up by a Madison Avenue adman. The word specifically refers to the psychological structure of the individual, and as such, it accurately describes my program of weight control which is built upon a mental, or psychological, approach to the cure of obesity.

We all have our own particular psychostructure, the formation and content of which determine our attitudes and outlook as well as our reaction to stimuli.

While everyone's psychostructure is different I discovered in a recent study of over twelve hundred obese patients that there are marked similarities among the psychostructures of men and women who suffer from overweight.

These similarities provided the key to formulation of guidelines to correct the compulsive eating habits of obese people, to help them restructure their responses so that undesirable urges can be overcome, thereby eliminating the major causes of their overweight condition.

To begin with, obese people, practically without exception, lead sedentary lives. Many of them have a mental aversion to exercise, and indulge in no daily exercise at all. No golf. No swimming. No walking. Their waking hours, for the most part, are spent sitting. They have never considered the idea of daily exercise, and even resist the idea. Their minds are programmed to *sit* instead of *move*. They tend to consider physical activity of any sort too much of an effort, and believe me, as a former 300 pounder, it *is* too great an effort! Yet they are all eager to lose weight, and express amazement when they are told that if they had walked a mile a day for the previous ten years, they would not have become overweight.

This was a startling revelation even to me. I had always believed that every human being was aware of the need for exercise to keep the body in shape. Obviously, there are many who don't, judging from the appalling number of overweight people in the world. It is interesting to note that in the last century, the caloric content of the American diet has actually diminished, yet today you have to hunt for the thin men and women while, a century ago, it was rare to see a fat person despite the fact that the diet in those days was higher in calories.

I also discovered that all the obese patients I examined were uniformly unable to resist external stimuli. They lacked the basic internal control mechanism which says "no" to certain foods and to second helpings. They were structured to reach out instead of refuse, even if they *knew* that certain foods would inevitably result in extra pounds.

This disclosure was reinforced by a series of experiments conducted by Dr. Shackner of some years ago that were specifically intended to determine the varying reactions of thin and fat people to external stimuli.

Believing they would be taking a written psychological test, a group of men and women were gathered in a classroom before noon time. Some of them were fat; some were thin. All had been requested to remove their wrist watches some time prior to the meeting, so their only means of knowing the time was a clock on the wall.

The group was unaware of two things: first, the clock on the wall had been advanced an hour; and second, the proposed written psychological test was merely an excuse. The real purpose of the experiment was to determine and assess any variance between the reactions of the thin and fat people towards the approach of an anticipated mealtime. In this case, lunch.

As the hands of the clock approached the noon hour, the fat members of the group began complaining of hunger. The thin members expressed no such desire for food.

The experiment was repeated a second time on a following day, but the clock was put *back* an hour instead of ahead. When the hands pointed to eleven o'clock, the fat subjects showed no reaction to the time, yet the thin people began experiencing hunger pains.

The conclusion was a significant revelation: the fat subjects' desire for lunch stemmed from their reaction to what the clock told them. In the first experiment, they *thought* it was lunchtime and became hungry; but they felt no such promptings in the second experiment because they *thought* it was only eleven o'clock.

The thin people, on the other hand, were unaffected by the false time on the clock, and only became hungry when their normal need for food told them it was time to eat.

These experiments were carried a step further: the same group was assembled and sandwiches were placed in open view in the classroom, with the invitation to partake if they felt hungry. The fat men and women helped themselves at once, whereas the thin subjects refrained.

Again the experiment was repeated but this time the sandwiches were placed out of sight in a refrigerator. At the end of the test, very few of the fat students had eaten a sandwich.

From this second set of experiments, it was concluded that the compulsive desire to eat in fat people stems from their reaction to external stimuli. When they *saw* the sandwiches displayed openly, they were unable to resist going forward and taking the food. When the sandwiches were concealed from view, the impulse to eat did not occur. *Out of sight, out of mind . . .*

With the thin people it made no difference. They were unaffected by the presence or absence of the food, and only ate when they were genuinely hungry.

And finally, a fairly common (though not universal) characteristic shared by obese men and women is a lack of assertiveness, which, when recognized by the individual, leads to feelings of frustration, anger, and emptiness. Failure to obtain normal gratification from life leads to an excessive dependence upon food as an alternate compensation.

These three common traits in obese people—a sedentary lifestyle, a lack of an internal control mechanism against external stimuli, and a lack of assertiveness—all contribute to an individual becoming overweight. It becomes clear that obesity is the *consequence* of certain conditions and habits in a person's life.

The reason for the failure of any attempt to lose weight permanently, lies in the common practice of treating the consequence rather than the cause.

Many doctors are guilty of making this mistake. They prescribe a diet supplemented by some medication. The patient dutifully loses twenty pounds, but within a short time after going "off" the diet and the medication will regain the weight. Why?

The patient has not altered his former habits and lifestyle which were the basic cause of his putting on the weight in the first place.

So he returns to his doctor, and they repeat the process again . . . and again . . . until eventually both the doctor and the patient become disgusted and totally discouraged and the patient resigns himself to being forever fat.

This syndrome of failure is precisely why there are so many overweight people despite their occasional attempts to reduce their weight. Until a person alters his habits through psychostructure, his obesity will continue to be a problem.

We've discussed the *cause* and the *consequence* of obesity. Now we must turn our attention to the *reaction,* or the effect of obesity upon the individual. Again, I found there are three major reactions to becoming overweight.

The first reaction is *depression.*

Psychiatrists generally classify depression in two categories: reactive and involutional.

Involutional depression is a serious problem and is often

treated with anti-depressant medication. Frequently the cause of this condition cannot be specifically pinpointed.

Reactive depression, on the other hand, is the result of a known cause, such as a death in the family, or a major financial or emotional setback. To cure this condition, the cause must be removed, or alternatively, the person must adjust to the situation.

The most common treatment of reactive depression is for a doctor or psychiatrist to prescribe an anti-depressant medication. Obesity causes a reactive depression so while medication may help temporarily, it is doomed to failure in the long run since a depression caused by obesity will not subside until the weight diminishes.

Closely tied with the symptom of depression is an anxiety syndrome, which is very prevalent when a patient reaches a certain weight.

A feeling of panic surfaces when a person becomes convinced his weight is out of control and he is turning into a walking mountain of flab! He believes his life will never be the same again, and he sees no way out of his dilemma. He becomes nervous, jumpy, and has difficulty sleeping. Fears pile upon fears as he experiences a sense of approaching doom. All these negative emotions combine to produce yet another condition: a desire for isolation.

Most fat people get to a point where they feel they would like crawling into a corner and hiding out of embarrassment, and figuratively speaking, many of them do.

They are ashamed of their appearance. They are afraid of unkind remarks from unfeeling friends and they retreat from social contact.

Ultimately, in extreme cases, obese people will withdraw from society, which is just as unhealthy psychologically as obesity is physically.

Wallowing in self-pity in their self-imposed isolation, obese men and women turn to their only remaining comfort: food, which, of course, only further compounds and exaggerates their problem.

This vicious cycle underlines the need for treating obesity from a psychological as well as a physical standpoint, which is exactly what psychostructure does.

A good illustration to this aspect of treatment is found in the case of Kenneth V., one of my patients. When he first arrived at my clinic, he was thirty-two years of age, five feet nine inches and weighed over 300 pounds. He said he was single and had never had a date with a girl in his life. Why? Because in college he had asked a girl out once, and she had refused, saying she wouldn't be seen in public with him. Kenneth knew he was fat, but he had never regarded himself as downright repulsive as the unfeeling coed had implied in her blunt refusal of his invitation.

Physical hurts can heal without trace, but psychological injuries can linger for a lifetime. So deeply did that girl's unkind remark affect Kenneth that he became shy, talking to women only when he had to in the course of his business, and then with an embarrassed mumble. His social life was minimal and his sex life non-existent.

Finally a friend suggested to Kenneth that he come to my clinic for treatment. When he began his program, his personality, understandably, was set: he was introspective and withdrawn. He remained in his room much of the time. At our regular group sessions, he sat quietly, observing but seldom participating. In the dining hall he ate alone at a separate table and left immediately after eating. Even in his personal counseling sessions, Kenneth rarely opened up—until he realized what was happening to him. He was *losing weight!* In fact, Kenneth V. is one of the most responsive patients I have ever treated. He lost more than a pound a day, and during the first month he lost forty-five pounds. With this fantastic response in his physique, came a positive mental response—in fact, almost a radical transformation! By the time Kenneth had shed over one hundred pounds, he was associating with other patients at the clinic, carrying on animated conversations, and reacting to his environment in a normal fashion instead of like a scared rabbit.

Kenneth left the clinic weighing 165 pounds, looking and sounding like a totally different person from the miserable, obese individual he had been on his arrival. His psychological change was almost as startling as his physical transformation.

He telephoned me a few weeks later, sounding almost incoherently happy. He had met a young woman and they had begun seeing each other regularly. Thirty-two might be a late age for a man to discover girls, but Kenneth made up for lost time. Thanks to his newly acquired normal physique and his blossoming personality, he was never without female company and made the most of his opportunities. He confessed he would never again let himself deteriorate into obesity, and he is successfully maintaining his daily diet and exercise routine to prevent any repetition of his former unhappy state.

As you restructure your attitudes, you will be able to regard food in its proper perspective—not as a source of solace, but of nutrition, to be taken in the right amounts and only when needed.

You will be able to enjoy your food without any sense of guilt and without feeling what you eat will add to your obesity.

Through psychostructure, you will be *in control* of what you eat, which is, first and foremost, the essential starting point in any effective effort to lose weight permanently.

Remember the Second Commandment of Psychostructure: *I will lose weight permanently as soon as I get rid of the cause of my overeating—out of sight, out of mind!*

3. HUNGER VS. APPETITE

"**D**on't ask me to cut down on eating," is a common plea I've heard over and over again, followed by, *"I'm always feeling hungry."*

Before starting your program of psychostructure you must understand that there is an important difference between hunger and appetite since much of your success will depend on your ability to recognize when you are *truly* hungry.

Hunger is the direct result of a definite physiological demand for food. When you feel truly hungry, you are experiencing the signals sent out by your system when nutrition is required for the continued maintenance of your bodily functions.

Not so with your appetite, which is more often than not prompted by some external stimulus that appeals to your senses rather than your basic bodily demand for food.

For example, you have just had dinner and as you take the dishes into the kitchen, you see a bar of chocolate on the shelf. Your taste buds immediately start to tingle as you recall your last piece of chocolate: creamy-rich, smooth, with an enticing flavor and tempting taste.

Your mouth starts to water, and your entire body yearns to have that succulent morsel enclosed in your mouth, slowly dissolving as you chew, then slipping down into your stomach with a final gulp of gustatory gratification.

Before you realize what you're doing, you reach out, strip off the the wrapper and pop the chocolate between your lips, and stand back, perhaps with your eyes closed, as you concentrate on that moment of pure delight.

You give not a single thought to the fact that you have just finished your dinner, have consumed possibly more food than you really needed and are feeling as full as the proverbial tick! Above all, you don't stop to consider the number of calories in the chocolate bar! You know only that for one single delicious moment, you are giving yourself over to pure eating enjoyment. Perhaps unconscious memories flood back from childhood when your mother promised you a piece of chocolate if you ate all your dinner . . . or washed behind your ears . . . or kept quiet for ten minutes. . . . You have reacted to years of prior programming that tell you a chocolate bar is something special—a reward —that spells exquisite enjoyment. Your reactions to the bar of chocolate have been so automatic that they could be called involuntary. You reached out because you couldn't help yourself—an excellent example of the power of your pre-conditioned psychostructure.

And don't underestimate the power of advertising that panders to the temptations of your appetite responses. Remember the drive-in restaurant, *Der Wienerschnitzel,* which has a very persuasive television commercial with a catch musical jingle that proclaims interminably: "Just thinking about those hot dogs makes you hungry." How appropriate is the use of that word "thinking"—but how inaccurate is the inclusion of the word "hungry."

The key to controlling your obesity lies in the *mind,* and the restructuring of your mental responses. In short, your *thoughts.*

Thinking about those hot dogs may make you want to rush out to the nearest *Wienerschnitzel* which is, of course, the prime purpose of the commercial.

But, to be technically correct, thinking about those hot dogs doesn't make you *hungry;* it merely stimulates your *appetite* and creates a strong desire for food that you may not really need.

If you are *truly* hungry (maybe you haven't eaten for six hours), then your response would be a valid one, the result of your bodily demand for nourishment; but if your body doesn't happen to *need* any food at that moment, that hot dog will only constitute additional calories and carbohydrates that will eventually surface as excess flab, no matter what your weight may be.

Remember that true hunger only occurs when you have been without food for a period of time and you begin to register certain internal physiological symptoms, one of the most common being extreme fatigue.

Remember that appetite stimulation occurs as a result of outside influences: seeing appealing foods, sweets or soft drinks, as well as smelling an odor that is tempting, like a cake baking in the oven.

There is only one cause of appetite stimulation that is not strictly mental, and it occurs when your blood sugar level drops. Let me explain how this happens so you can guard against giving in to this urge when and if it should occur.

When a person eats a meal high in carbohydrates, the blood sugar rises quickly to a high level. To compensate for this unnatural condition, the pancreas discharges a large amount of insulin which lowers the blood sugar again. However, in the course of this process, there is a stimulation of the appetite, which is the reason why many people feel the desire to eat within a short time after having a meal. Remember, if this urge is ignored, the feeling will disappear in a short time as the body adjusts itself to a normal blood sugar level.

If you do *not* ignore this condition, and consume more food, you will only trigger the same sequence: the blood sugar will rise quickly; the pancreas will put out more insulin; the blood sugar will come down and you will experience a repetition of the desire to eat . . . another of the vicious cycles that are particularly hazardous for someone suffering from overweight, because the more you give in to such symptoms, the more food you will be shoveling into your stomach, and the more you will be adding to your obesity. This repeated eating is an example of the power of positive reinforcement. You have an uncomfortable feeling—you eat—the feeling leaves. But because you responded positively to the feeling by eating, the feeling will be more likely to return.

So if you have your dinner at seven o'clock, and then feel a craving for a snack at eleven, turn your back on the refrigerator, and go to bed! The desire to eat will probably disappear by the time you fall asleep, and you'll be that many more calories ahead of the game.

Being able to distinguish between feeling truly hungry and experiencing appetite stimulation does not automatically mean that if you eat only when you are truly hungry you will not derive any pleasure or get any satisfaction from your meals. Far from it. A thin person who eats mainly when he feels the need for bodily nourishment may certainly enjoy his food, just as you, an overweight person, can enjoy and feel fully satisfied with simple meals once you have restructured and reprogrammed yourself to look upon eating as a means of providing essential nourishment to your body rather than as an abnormal means of sensual gratification.

In fact, all the positive appetite responses which have caused and continue to compound your obesity can be overcome through psychostructure. Your present appetite for fattening foods will be eliminated from your mind, enabling your body to return to, and retain a normal weight.

It is a matter of *attitude*—the result of mental responses to stimuli that are followed by an undesirable reaction. You will learn that ten percent of the problem of obesity is physical (your diet) while ninety percent is mental (your innate psychostructure). Why do you think so many overweight people fail in their efforts to reduce? They may be on a perfectly valid diet that would, in time, lower their weight, but they lack the mental capacity to stick to it. They become impatient (a common condition when you realize weight loss does not occur overnight) and they become disgusted with their progress, then discouraged, and then they give up!

Which underlines the critical necessity for adopting a positive attitude towards losing weight. Don't ever believe you won't be able to do it; because you *can,* and you *will,* just like thousands of others who have followed the psychostructure program faithfully, every step of the way, no matter how insignificant some of the directives may appear to be.

Just as you may not have been aware of the difference between hunger and appetite, so also must you draw a line between your total desired weight loss and your weekly goal.

To concentrate on the numerical figure you plan to lose in order to achieve the physical figure you desire can be traumatic; for example, the idea of having to lose 150 pounds can be pretty scary, especially if you have tried before and failed.

That was exactly the problem with Mrs. Betty Hughes, wife of the former governor of New Jersey. She came to me in November of 1975 after exhausting many other possibilities. She tried hypnosis, Dr. Atkins, Dr. Stillman, fasting, all with some successful loss, followed by a rapid gain. She very successfully completed nineteen weeks on the Kempner rice diet on which she lost 80 pounds that she kept off for one year. But by 1973 she was again 125 pounds overweight. Completely discouraged, she arranged for an ileal bypass, with tragic results. After the operation she experienced diarrhea, vomiting, hair loss, nausea, bleeding gums, and total dehydration. Nine months after the operation she was down to 134 pounds but she also had liver damage and a total imbalance of blood components, which led to admission at a Princeton New Jersey hospital, where her condition deteriorated to a comotose state. She was rushed in an ambulance to Massachusettes General. Following six weeks of internal feeding, ileal bypass reversal was performed.

Mrs. Hughes remained hospitalized for nine weeks, needing round the clock nursing care. Within a year she had regained sixty pounds, at which time she weighed 218. By June of 1974, she was tipping the scales at her all-time high of 236.5 When she came to me in November of 1975, the 54-year-old Mrs. Hughes, aside from being obese was tearful, depressed and arthritic. She checked into my clinic and eight months later (July, 1976) she was 100 pounds lighter, her depression eliminated, arthritis under control. This loss has been maintained with minimal difficulty, and Mrs. Hughes now lectures at the clinic on a part-time basis during her reinforcement visits. Her happiness with the program is expressed in her own words below:

I feel better than I have in thirty years! The weight loss, of course, was a great help to my morale. More importantly, I have learned for the first time that I have an incurable disease that can be controlled! Dr. Stuelke's program is at last a realistic approach to a long-term problem.

If you set a goal of a pound a week, or two pounds a week, whichever you decide upon, this becomes psychologically reassuring because it's a goal you feel confident you can reach. In my psychostructure program, weight losses of three to five pounds a week are not uncommon. Then as each week passes, and your bathroom scale tells you the good news, the feeling of accomplishment will spur you on, will add to your self-confidence, and will reaffirm and increase your determination to succeed, no matter how long it takes. Never dwell upon your *total* objective. Live one day at a time, and lose weight one day at a time!

Remember a journey starts with the first step, and is completed one step at a time. The more weight you have to lose, the more vital it is not to let the idea of your total weight loss discourage you, which it assuredly will if you brood over it too much.

I knew one man who wanted to lose 180 pounds which is, admittedly, a tremendous amount. When he had only dropped fifty pounds in six months, he grew very discouraged and gave up. He failed to realize that his excessive overweight had built up in his body over a period of ten years; yet he felt thwarted at not being able to lose it in six months! Fortunately for himself, this man started my program of psychostructure and succeeded eventually; it took him almost two years, but he confessed afterwards that he never once became discouraged because he learned to approach the program day by day, enjoying his successful weight loss pound by pound.

I also remember William J., who was 150 pounds overweight when he came to my clinic. His physical condition was appalling. He could barely walk. His attitude alternated from impulsive anger to pitiful indecision. His story was truly a sad one, but an excellent example of how obesity can creep up and take over a person's life before he realizes what is happening.

William J. owns and operates one of the largest trucking firms in the south. Some years ago when the economy began slipping, William's business began falling off. As he saw his income diminishing he became concerned, then frustrated, and depressed. Without realizing it, he began venting his frustrations at the dinner table. He ate more and more, and began putting on weight. He found himself becoming indecisive at times; then he would have periods of aggression. He fired many of his staff on the spur of the moment, foolishly letting people go at a time when he needed them. As his business began to flounder, he found himself eating more, until one day he realized how obese he had become; but by then, it was too late. He was caught in a vicious cycle of his own making. The worse his business became, the more he ate, and the fatter he got. The fatter he got, the less attention he paid to his business. The less attention he paid to his business the more it failed; the more business failed, the more he ate. Finally, he abandoned all attempts to save his firm, and realized that something had to be done about his physical condition, which by then was completely out of hand.

He came to my clinic and began his program of psychostructure. He remained a patient at the clinic until he had lost 150 pounds, by which time he was not only once more in good physical shape, but his mental approach to life also had undergone a complete transformation.

Despite the changing economic climate, he realized that most of his business reverses had been the result of his own mismanagement and poor judgment. He returned to his work and began rebuilding his life and his business. His renewed enthusiasm and energy had their effect. Gradually he was able to salvage what was left; begin a fresh, assertive effort at running his trucking firm.

Today, William's business is thriving, and he himself is active, energetic, and successful—not only as a businessman, but as an obesity-prone individual who had learned to restructure his lifestyle in order to control his weight.

Understandably every obese person wonders how long it will take before he can achieve a normal body weight and start enjoying a normal life again. A year . . . two years . . . what does it matter? You do it, step by step, and however long it takes, that period is insignificant compared with a lifetime of obesity. (However, to some extent, I will satisfy your curiosity: most of my very obese patients have been able to lose their total desired number of pounds within a year!)

I must emphasize the difference between my program of psychostructure and a "diet." My program does not merely mean "going on a diet" and restricting your food intake for a certain period of time.

Psychostructure is a *lifetime* program of weight control. By adhering to the program, you will be able to lose weight and keep it off permanently. You will be following a structured diet, but once you reach your desired weight, you do not deviate from this diet—you can merely increase the amount. If you stick to the right foods, you will not regain weight, and by that time, believe me, you will be psychologically reprogrammed so that you won't even consider reaching for the wrong foods!

Remember the Third Commandment of Psychostructure: *I will not dwell on my intended total weight loss but will take one day at a time just as I will lose one pound at a time.*

4. FACTS ABOUT FOOD AND EXERCISE

Food and exercise are essential for bodily survival, but the shape we survive in depends in large measure on the type and quantity of food we eat and the amount of exercise we have. It is impossible to lose excess weight and maintain a healthy body without monitoring both food and exercise and making sure you get the right amounts of each; not occasionally, but every day of your life.

Do I hear groans of disapproval? Fine. I've heard these before, many times. Where does disapproval originate? In the mind, of course—which only proves my point: that to be permanently successful at controlling your weight, you have to alter your attitudes, to restructure yourself to look upon sensible eating and exercise as daily essentials in maintaining your normal weight and health. Believe me, this is no hardship. The diet I prescribe places no strain upon your enjoyment of your meals. The exercise I insist upon is neither time-consuming nor strenuous; yet even if it were, is not a few minutes of effort a day preferable to years of misery being overweight?

You *do* have to exercise, and you *do* have to restrict your diet. Let's talk about those few certain foods which must be eliminated if you are going to lose weight.

First, high carbohydrate foods with a high sugar content must be avoided. Just as salt causes the body to retain fluids, so also do carbohydrates result in fluid retention, because fluid is necessary to dissolve carbohydrates before they can be burned.

People who have followed one of the carbohydrate diets often find their weight increasing out of proportion to the calories consumed. This is due to the fluid retention properties of carbohydrates. Since this is a fact of life, there is nothing you can do about it, except keep away from carbohydrates.

As you learned in the last chapter, carbohydrates which are high in sugar also have the undesirable effect of stimulating the appetite due to the hypoglycemic response of the body—the pancreas putting out insulin to lower the increase in blood sugar, which in turn causes appetite stimulation.

Foods that contain a great amount of sugar and starch should be avoided, not only during your initial period of weight loss, but afterwards as well to prevent gaining the weight back.

The oldest form of food in the world is also one of the most weight producing: bread, and it is one of the major causes of obesity today. Think about this: no one ever takes a single slice by itself. Bread is always eaten in addition to other foods, never as a substitute for them. The majority of people eat around eight slices a day. That's about 500 calories that slip into the system, not counting the calories contained in whatever is spread on the bread. Beware of the breads that claim to "build bodies twelve ways," because one of the ways is *sideways!*

Eliminating bread from your diet entirely would put you fifty pounds ahead each year, to say nothing of bypassing the calories contained in the items we ladle so liberally on top of bread: butter, jelly, mayonnaise, cheese, gravy and such. But more about the dangers of bread later.

Concentrated foods should also be avoided: items that appear small in size but which are high in calories, such as butter or cheese. One teaspoon of butter, for example, contains forty-five calories.

The most significant drawback of concentrated foods stems from the inability of most obese people to gauge a portion correctly. Given the same size portions of food, a thin person will overestimate the amount, but a fat person will underestimate—making him take more than he should for a serving. One dip of ice cream looks big to a thin person, small to a fat person.

An essential part of the psychostructure program is policing not only the type but also the amount of food you consume. Concentrated items, therefore, constitute a potential danger because of your inherent inaccuracy in judging the amount you put on your plate.

Advertising is primarily responsible for another major dietary hazard for American adults: milk. The rest of the world gets by very well without it, but here, thanks to the millions spent by the American Dairy Association, we have been brainwashed into believing that milk is "nature's most perfect food." It is—but only for baby cows!

For the average adult, three glasses of whole milk each day will add at least twenty-five pounds to your body weight in a year. Eliminating the accustomed glass of milk with your meals will go a long way in cutting down your overweight condition and keeping off excess pounds.

The problem is focused in our basic attitude towards milk. Most people regard it as a *drink,* and use it to quench their thirst. Milk is, however, a *food,* and swallowing one glass of whole milk means you've poured more than one hundred calories into your system when a glass of water or unsweetened iced tea would quench your thirst without adding the calories.

Along with milk, sugared soft drinks are liquids to be avoided. The average regular soft drink contains around 125 calories per bottle. If you're a cola or an un-cola freak, I suggest you switch to the non-calorie type which contains as few as two calories per glassful.

As a general rule, if you eliminate bread; foods that are high in sugar; concentrated foods such as butter and cheese; milk, and sugared soft drinks, you can eat just about anything else you want without endangering your weight.

In fact, if you eliminate bread and milk from your diet and

walk two miles a day, you will find your body weight declining to its natural level and never be bothered with obesity again. Is this too dangerously simple a statement? To some it may be, but it happens to be true. As the late Adele Davis said many times, "We are what we eat."

Another vital factor in weight control is *your attitude,* which is why I took the calculated risk in saying above that cutting out bread and milk and walking two miles a day would solve your problem! I know from experience that very few, if any, would be able to do this! They may start out full of high hopes and unbending ambition, but without changing their basic attitudes (which is what you do in the program of psychostructure), they will inevitably revert back to their old, weight producing routine.

Just as attitude is important in regard to your choice of food, so also is it crucial in regard to exercise. As I said before, no diet can be totally successful without including some form of daily exercise.

The usual resistance to exercise stems from the idea that it has to be arduous, unpleasant, and exhausting. Not so. Don't think I'm going to recommend an hour in the gym lifting heavy weights! Weight lifting is for weight lifters, and certainly should be avoided by anyone suffering from obesity.

I recommend only simple exercising of the body. Excessive strain and strenuous exercise routines can place undue pressures on the heart and musculoskeletal systems, and who would welcome the idea of losing weight at the expense of suffering a coronary or severe aches and pains.

I have found that many people disregard exercise because they consider it unimportant. *Why* is exercise essential? Because it constitutes a natural means of burning away fat, or utilizing energy. The two are synonymous.

Your body uses energy in breathing; in maintaining its temperature; in conducting the many processes inherent in the system; even in keeping your heart beating. Just as our modern civilization depends on energy, or oil, to keep the wheels of progress turning, so also does the body need energy for its survival. Just as we store oil in the basement for winter heating, so also does the body store energy for those moments when it is needed.

When you do not use up sufficient energy each day, you start accumulating fat. Does this mean you have to start leading a very active life? Not at all. You merely have to start walking, starting with as little as a block a day and increasing your distance gradually as you feel up to it, and you *will* begin to feel up to it!

A word of advice: just as I said before about taking one day at a time in setting your weight-loss goal, so also take one step at a time. I knew one person who decided if one mile was good, ten miles would be better! He wound up with blisters, utter exhaustion, and couldn't walk again for two weeks. Start by walking a realistic distance. As you lose weight and your endurance increases, you can walk as far as you want to, and feel you are capable of doing so without overtiring yourself.

You can walk anywhere, anytime. One word of caution, however, for people living in snow country. The heart is subject to extreme stress from exercising in cold weather. The reason is that cold air entering the lungs causes constriction of the arteries, resulting in less oxygen getting into the system. How often have we all read about deaths caused by a sudden snowstorm where the strain of shoveling snow has brought on a heart attack? If your body's in top shape, naturally there is less danger, but most people who try to clear the sidewalk after a snowstorm are usually not in condition for such strenuous activity. So take it easy in cold weather. You can still enjoy your daily walk, but don't overdo it!

When should you walk? Anytime you're able and feel like it, but the best time for reinforcing your weight reduction is after a meal. As I mentioned earlier, the body temperature rises after eating; this thermal response is caused by the actual digestion of your food, a process that is prolonged by exercise, resulting in a greater consumption of calories. Because the evening meal is usually the largest meal of the day, I recommend a walk after dinner each night, though any time is acceptable.

If you are not used to walking very much, make sure that you have a comfortable, good fitting pair of shoes to prevent the possibility of blisters. A combination of a cotton and nylon sock (nylon on the inside and cotton on the outside) helps to prevent friction between your feet and your shoes, especially in winter when you may be wearing heavier socks that sometimes tend to wrinkle up and cause blisters.

Walking should be done at a comfortable pace. There is an insignificant difference between the energy consumption walking a mile slowly and walking more briskly. However, if you walk for a solid hour at a fast clip, you will burn more energy than if you amble along; but that is a difference based on *time* not distance. For the purposes of completing your required walking for your weight-loss program, the *distance* should be the determining factor, irrespective of how fast you complete your walk.

Of course, there are other forms of exercise: such as tennis, golf, swimming, skiing, bowling. If you can indulge in these, so much the better, but I have recommended walking, not only because it is a proven aid in losing weight, but because it takes nothing more than putting on your shoes and getting out of the house. You can do it anywhere, almost anytime. No special equipment is needed. You don't have to have a partner or join an expensive health club and you don't have to worry about a certain time to do it. Walking is just about the only exercise that is available, free, to everyone.

In addition to helping you lose weight, walking is highly beneficial for people suffering from hypertension and coronary artery disease. People with psychological and nervous problems will find an immediate improvement after beginning a program of walking every day. Cholesterol levels also drop, which is another beneficial side effect of walking, or of any exercise done regularly.

Some people who enjoy exercise often neglect this important facet of well-being after they become overweight. Sandra M. was such a woman—basically an outdoor type, she had kept her weight under control by weekly exercise; but when she was put on a special assignment by her firm that required her working ten hours a day, weekends included, she let her frequent tennis and swimming sessions drop. In three months she had gone from a slender, attractive young woman to someone definitely fat. Not just overweight, but *fat!* To make her condition even more unbearable, Sandra was a beautiful woman. As the fat started creeping up, her exquisite features became submerged beneath layers of flab. When Sandra realized what had happened, she began losing her self-esteem. Her special work was to continue for another three months, and she literally gave up.

As is quite common with women who begin putting on excess weight, Sandra began losing interest in her appearance. She was careless about her dress. Her hair became untidy and her makeup was minimal. Like so many others in the same predicament, she didn't care how she looked. She had the attitude that she was fat, nobody wanted her, so why bother?

She told me frankly that since she had put on so much weight, she had quit buying fashionable clothes (No woman looks good in a size 18, she said disgustedly) and bought large, tent-type mumus that covered as much of her body as possible. She couldn't remember when she had her hair done last, and her face was devoid of makeup. In short, she had turned into a slob, despite the fact that beneath those rolls of fat there lay a truly beautiful face.

Slowly, as she began to lose weight, she began taking a little pride in her appearance once again. She started fixing her hair, and using makeup. Watching this young woman each day was like observing a flower slowly opening, until the total beauty was again revealed.

As well as going on a restricted diet, Sandra began once more indulging in daily exercise—not only the walking which I prescribe, but swimming and tennis. When Sandra left the clinic, she wore a skimpy halter and a pair of brief tennis shorts. Her bare midriff was symbolic of the change that had occurred in her. Not only was her body in terrific shape but her face also glowed radiantly and her spirits were obviously soaring. She told me she had learned her lesson: she would remain on a restricted diet and maintain her weekly exercise schedule as before, and never again allow herself to become overweight. She walked out not only with the right *body,* but the right *attitude* towards her body and what she put into it at mealtimes.

Some health clubs claim that they have machines that will "spot reduce." *Totally* untrue! A strange rotating machine may buffet your bottom until you're blue, but the only way you'll reduce your derriere is by reducing your overall body weight.

Why? Because when your body starts losing weight, it loses it *all over* in keeping with the way your fat is spread over your body, a condition that is genetically determined. Remember the three basic physical types we described earlier? Fat or thin, you belong in one of these types, and no amount of dieting or exercise will ever change your basic physical type.

You cannot lose off your hips without losing proportionately elsewhere. If you are especially anxious to reduce the size of your hips (a major disaster area with many obese women), you will find your face, your arms and your legs diminishing in size along with your hips. There's no way to "spot reduce," so don't ever let yourself be talked into wasting money at places or on elaborate devices that claim this to be possible. Too many people are *seduced* by advertising claims instead of being *reduced* by proper professional weight-loss methods. I recall one woman who first thought she could "spot reduce" at a health club.

Joan R. is a housewife in her mid-twenties with two children. Today she and her husband are enjoying their marriage, consummating their mutual feelings of love and respect, and building a future together. But their home was not always a happy one, as I learned from the family doctor who referred her case to me.

Joan had begun putting on weight after the birth of her children. As most mothers are aware, weight increase often occurs during pregnancy, which is why diet control is always advisable for pregnant women. Some women will revert to their normal weight after giving birth, but there are those, like Joan, who do not. She began getting larger and larger, and with her mounting obesity, she started suffering from insomnia. Her sexual relations with her husband deteriorated until they were almost non-existent. She imagined he was having an affair with his secretary, because of his lack of interest in her sexually. She failed to understand that he was no longer stimulated because, in fact, he found her repulsive. At this time, Joan was grossly overweight, a tragic contrast to the slender woman that had walked down the aisle ten years before.

She quit buying new clothes, making the excuse that there was only money enough for the children's wardrobe. She stopped wearing makeup, and began deteriorating physically and mentally.

She became subject to intense fits of depression, weeping often and interminably, spilling forth her sad story to anyone willing to listen. Finally, after almost four years, she went to her family doctor in a state of suicidal depression. The following week she was admitted to my clinic and began the slow road back to physical and mental health once more.

Joan responded well. Obviously (and this is common with people who have been obese for years) she had reached the end of her capacity to tolerate her condition. She followed my program religiously, and began to lose weight very quickly. After losing her first forty pounds, she went to the beauty parlor for the first time in four years. She took a rewarding interest in her facial appearance and began carefully using makeup. She expressed an interest in taking up tennis and golf, both of which naturally supplemented her daily exercise routine of walking. By this time, her fits of depression were a thing of the past, and she was exhibiting a healthy mental outlook towards herself, and towards others.

Joan completed her program and returned home a totally new and different woman. She resumed normal sexual relations with her husband to the great satisfaction of them both. She started taking dancing lessons and began making new social contacts. For the first time in four years, she was able to look at herself in the mirror without cringing. Her self-esteem and self-confidence were restored to a remarkable degree.

Today she is not only physically in top shape, but is admirably adjusted psychologically. Aware of what might happen again if she lets herself go, she still limits her meals and makes sure she gets daily exercise. She has restructured her lifestyle successfully, a change which she realizes is essential to maintain the happiness of both herself and her family.

Like many obese people who are disproportionately large in certain areas such as the hips or the legs, Joan became somewhat discouraged during the first weeks of her weight-loss program. She saw herself losing weight, but those certain extra-fat areas still remained extra-large. As I said, there is no such thing as "spot reducing"; as the body loses weight, it loses it all over, and every patient undertaking a weight-loss program should realize that if you achieve the ideal weight for your height and age, you can only be grateful that you have conquered your obesity. But if your normal, natural figure (as genetically determined) contains hips or legs that are a little larger than average, you just have to learn to accept this, just as you must accept your height, shoe size, and skin color. We are what we are—and only if we are *fat* can we ever hope to change ourselves into a more appealing shape. But change the way our bodies are basically constructed—never! Learning to accept ourselves is always a big step in cultivating that needed feeling of self-esteem, especially after losing excess fat that has hidden our real selves beneath those layers of flab!

So remember: losing weight will help you achieve a normal healthy body, with everything in proportion for your particular physical type—but you will never alter your basic physiological structure.

Don't feel discouraged at this point if you *are* resisting the idea of having to restrict your diet and having to exercise every day.

After all, if you hadn't been adverse to such a regimen all these years, you wouldn't be overweight now, would you? Let's not brood over past failures, which only reinforce your negative outlook towards losing weight. Accentuate the positive. *Believe,* not just in this program, but in *yourself* and your ability to succeed.

You want to lose weight, don't you? Very well. The next chapter tells you how.

Remember the Fourth Commandment of Psychostructure: *I will eat three carefully balanced meals a day and I will walk whenever and wherever I can.*

5. RESTRUCTURING YOUR LIFESTYLE

You will recall from the previous chapters how it was established through various experiments and observations that thin people have some type of internal self-regulating mechanism which controls their eating habits, which an obese person lacks.

Simply, a thin person is not prone to obesity because he doesn't overeat, while those suffering from overweight bring on their problem and compound it by reaching out instead of refusing. . . . Does this mean that if a thin person were forcibly stuffed with food, he would gain weight? Possibly, but it just doesn't happen.

The internal control mechanism guards a thin person against any unwise and unplanned consumption of food. He may be surrounded by tempting delicacies, and he may nibble a morsel or two, but he doesn't gorge himself uncontrollably like most fat people are prone to do. His internal control mechanism is his guardian angel!

For an obese person to achieve this type of control, therefore

(I call it control, but a better word might be instinct)—he has to consciously control his environment, not only during the time he is restructuring his mental responses, but as a permanent safeguard against falling back into bad habits.

How can I possibly control my environment, you ask. First, by keeping food out of sight and out of reach, which means a basic change in your lifestyle.

Does this sound impossible? Maybe at first, but not after you learn how. For example, you may work in an office, where the usual routine involves coffee and rolls being brought in at ten each morning. If you are not in a position to prevent this, make it your business to leave until the morning coffee break is over. I mean it! Get up from your desk, go to the water cooler and have a glass of water if you like. But whatever happens, get yourself away from that tempting aroma and those delicious looking donuts and sweet rolls, because if you don't, you're going to find yourself reaching out and consuming over 200 calories before you realize it, and you'll be guilty of *unstructured* eating. Coffee and donuts are *not* part of your diet; therefore they have no business in your life; and if you can't *see* them, you're not going to be tempted to *eat* them. Out of sight, out of mind . . .

This is a simple example of an important part in restructuring your lifestyle, especially when starting out on my program. Eventually you may accomplish the instinctive resistance that seems to be inherent in a naturally thin person, but until you do, it is vitally important that you take every possible step to control your environment, to change the world around you as much as you can to prevent having your appetite stimulated by the sight and smell of food, and even the *sound* of cooking! If there is ice cream in your freezer, you are going to eat it. If there are potato chips on the pantry shelf, you are going to eat them. The sooner you admit this fact, the closer you will come to accepting the idea that a basic change is required to help you control your diet.

Environmental structuring is a unique concept when it comes to the treatment of obesity, and I have established it as the only method that will guarantee a permanent solution to your weight problem. You have quite possibly tried other methods before, most of which direct their efforts towards the individual. "Take these pills." "Eat only these foods." "Drink eighty ounces of water each day." Such directives deal only with the symptoms—fat—and not with the cause, which, among other things, is your environment and your reaction to external stimuli.

I can suggest many ways to help, but you will have to analyze your daily routine and list those places and situations that you are going to *have* to avoid. The success of any system of weight control depends more on the *patient* than the doctor. So also in this phase of psychostructure: you have to cooperate once you know what is expected of you; and I expect you to start making a list right away of danger spots each day in your life.

If you pass a bakery or a delicatessen on your way to work each morning, change your route. If you think this isn't important, start adding up the number of times you *haven't* passed the bakery, but have walked in and bought a bundle of goodies to stash in your desk drawer for munching on between meals. You can't remember? Well, you *will* be remembering, because you are going to make a list of everything you eat, every day.

When you go out to eat, avoid buffet-line-type restaurants, and stay away from your favorite eating place that serves the best lasagna this side of Napoli. Even if you enjoy the atmosphere, you're going to be unable to sit there and order a salad when those enticing aromas are filling the air. Accept the fact that you are helpless in the face of temptation, so don't lay yourself wide open to any type of unstructured eating. You're going to be on a diet from now on, and if you shudder at the prospect, just keep thinking about that fabulous slender figure you're going to have in another few months. . . . Keep your mind on your objective. Resist any inclination to indulge yourself.

I won't dispute the undeniable fact that it is impossible to change the world. There will be many aspects of your environment that cannot be altered—unless, of course, you retreat to the mountains and become a hermit!

Then how do you deal with those temptations that you can't avoid? Simple, really: with intellectual, or *mind* control.

This is not to be confused with *self-control*, which, as we have already shown, an obese person unfortunately lacks. You may feel this is a put-down, and claim this isn't true with you. But if it wasn't, why are you overweight right now? Just as you look at your physical self in the mirror each day, so also must you look at your psychological self, and you must look *honestly*. No excuses. Admit it to yourself. You're fat. You may be *grossly* overweight. So let's do something about it, and get your mind on the right track so we can get your body down to its right weight once more.

There's more to this than merely changing your mind. As obese people lack the naturally thin person's internal mechanism that helps keep him from overeating, you have to replace that internal psychological mechanism with a means of combatting your instinctive desire to eat too much.

This is done by a technique called *documentation,* or the recording of significant information on a regular basis. How? With a daily diary and a weight chart. Therefore, you will not only *watch* what you eat, but you will *record everything* you eat, thereby giving you positive reinforcement each day that you are not slipping away from your new routine. Your weight chart, too, serves as a positive indication that your efforts are succeeding.

Let's go into this more fully so you will understand the reasons for and the advantages of documentation in relation to your decision to lose weight.

First, documentation provides absolute proof of your daily consumption of food. You will have your calories down in black and white so that there is no room for doubt over what you have or have not eaten.

Why is this so important? Because through research I have discovered that obese people simply do not have the capacity to judge their daily food consumption correctly. In actuality the obese person may be eating twice as much food as he or she *thought.*

When you are able to see written evidence, you will become intellectually aware of what you are eating, and be able to exercise control—or I should say you will *learn* to exercise control as you slowly become restructured mentally through the daily regimen of documentation.

Should you fall from grace and have a brief period of *unstructured* eating (you had an ice cream cone when you took the kids to the zoo!), you will see this on your daily record, and on reviewing your figures each night, as you should, there will be a negative reinforcement to your psychostructure, enabling you to rekindle your determination to avoid other possible periods of unstructured eating.

Documentation provides both negative and positive reinforcement. You saw an example of negative reinforcement in the preceding paragraph. Positive reinforcement is provided in your daily documentation by underlining the gains you make each day, and compared with your previous eating habits, sticking to the caloric limitations of your diet *is* a gain. Every day that your total consumption of food does not exceed the number of calories specified in your diet is cause for celebration.

But remember: never dwell on your *total* desired weight loss. Take each day at a time, and concern yourself only with your *weekly* weight loss.

Accordingly, when you review your documentation each night, look upon your written record as so many ounces or pounds you have lost. Give yourself a mental pat on the back for not indulging in any unstructured eating. Recall any incident where you stood firm and didn't give in to temptation, perhaps when a friend was eating a candy bar and offered you a bite—and you *refused*! Total success is made up of a multitude of minor victories like this. But again (and if I stress this point too much, there is a reason), such little victories are *mental,* showing that through repetition and firm resolve, you *are* reprogramming your responses, pushing your own psychostructure into a new pattern of behavior that excludes *any* food you are not supposed to have. Which is why I have stressed patience and perseverance as prerequisites to your success.

Let me give you an example of something very simple which will help you tremendously in avoiding the temptation of friends who try to entice you to eat when you are really not inclined to do so.

If you will observe your thin friends at a function where food is being offered, you will note the interesting phrase "No, thank you," being used repeatedly by thin people. Think back. Let your mind recall those parties in the past: how many times have you been offered food, and refused? I suspect there have been few times—very few times! As I've pointed out before, those of us with a weight problem lack the internal control mechanism that enables us to automatically refuse food when we are not really hungry.

As a daily exercise, practice saying "No, thank you," and the next time, at a gathering, or at work, or in a restaurant, when someone offers you food, just say "No, thank you," without thinking, without analyzing, without looking. Just say it! "NO, THANK YOU."

You will find this spontaneous response to food will come to you very easily after awhile, especially when you remind yourself afterwards the number of calories you're saving yourself.

One of the most positive reinforcements you will have will be your weight chart, with its steadily descending graph line that proves, day in and day out, that you are on your way to permanent weight control.

Proof of positive reinforcement from daily documentation came from one study I conducted at Duke University. Using a test group of 267 patients who were going through psychostructure at the Dietary Rehabilitation Clinic, I observed that those men and women who were most conscientious in maintaining daily records of their food and their weight proved to be the patients who achieved the greatest success in losing weight.

YOUR DAILY DIARY

There are ten important steps in the use of your daily diary.

ONE: Buy a small pocket notebook and designate this as your weight control diary. Print in block letters on the cover: WEIGHT CONTROL DIARY. Use this notebook for nothing else but a record of your progress. On the inside cover, note the date, month and year. Regard this date as the official beginning of your diet—the day that you definitely decide you are no longer going to be obese. You are on the threshold of a new life, and you must impress this on your consciousness, which will be a positive reinforcement for your psychostructure. Past failures mean nothing. Past indecision is forgotten. You have mentally turned from your old inhibiting ideas about yourself and look *forward* now, *not* back. You must discard any ideas of limitation from your mind. Nothing can hold you back now. You're on your way! *Believe* in your infinite capacity to succeed, in your own mental processes to strengthen your resolve to restructure your lifestyle, your attitudes, your outlook, and become the person you've always wanted to be—slender and healthy, enjoying life to the fullest in every way. You can do *anything* you set your mind to! Clear all past ideas from your mind so thoroughly that thoughts of your obesity will never cloud your consciousness, or deter your resolve. Remember, as often as you can, *you are going to succeed.* Make this a daily affirmation, especially as you use your diary to enter some information, which you will do every time you consume a morsel of food; every time you take any form of exercise. At the risk of being irreligious, I ask you to regard your diary as your Bible. Just as we gain daily strength from meditation on our faith, so will you gain daily inspiration and a sense of accomplishment from the record of your progress. Never regard your diary as a chore; rather look upon it as a welcome and essential part of your program to achieve the body weight you desire.

TWO: Carry your diary with you *at all times.* No matter how reliable you regard your memory, it's your enemy when it comes to remembering what you eat. Have that notebook handy every moment of your waking hours, no matter where you go or what you may be doing.

THREE: In addition to the date at the beginning of your diary, write in the day of the week, every day, for example: Monday, September 6.

FOUR: Under the date, add the number of days you have been following your diet. This number will naturally increase by one each day.

FIVE: On each page (one page per day is usual), allow space for you to write in the quantity and type of food for each meal, and divide this space into three: breakfast, lunch and dinner.

SIX: Calculate the number of calories consumed at each meal, and insert the figure after noting down the food eaten.

SEVEN: U.S.E. stands for "unstructured eating." Don't imagine you'll never indulge yourself outside your diet. You will, especially in the beginning; after all, you can't expect to be perfect right off the bat! For this reason, you should leave space on each page for any possible moments of unstructured eating.

Record not only what you ate and the number of calories involved, but the circumstances, such as (a) who you were with; (b) where you did the eating; (c) what time of the day it was; (d) how you were feeling at the time. The reason for this detail is that you will thereby be better able to analyze the situations, times, places, etc., when you became unstructured. For example, at the end of the week, you may notice that every time you met a certain friend at a particular restaurant, you joined him in a bite to eat. So . . . make a mental note to change your meeting place from a restaurant to some other location, and help yourself guard against any future unstructured eating episodes.

EIGHT: Record the number of structured miles you walk each day. Only *planned, structured* walking, remember! Strolling up to the market, or walking around the house should not be included.

NINE: Record exercise other than walking, such as tennis or swimming, and include the time involved.

TEN: At the bottom of each page, write in the total number of calories consumed each day.

As a guide, there follows a sample page from the diary used in my clinic by every patient enrolled in the program. Even though patients in my clinic get daily staff supervision in their program, they still have to fill out their own diary each day, just as you will be doing. Why? Because when you do it yourself, you are providing daily positive reinforcement of the principles of psychostructure, and helping *yourself* towards your ultimate goal.

Day_____ Date_____ Day No._____
FOODS

Bk.
 	
                              C_____
 	
L.
 	
                              C_____
 	
D.
 	
                              C_____

U.S.E. Who What When Where & How?
Total Calories
EXERCISE
Walk_____miles Other:

You will notice that in your daily diary, there is no place for recording your daily weight. This is because the diary is concerned only with those factors over which you exert direct control. The degree to which you are able to maintain such control will determine the amount of your weight loss, which is recorded in your weight chart. In your diary, you record only your diet and your exercise, which is all you should think about when you take it out of your pocket to make an entry. Worrying about your rate of weight loss can be psychologically inhibiting. Just know (*be-*

lieve!) that if you follow your program conscientiously, your weight *will* diminish, as it assuredly will if you confine yourself only to structured eating.

YOUR WEIGHT CHART

I've yet to meet an obese person who doesn't have a scale in his or her bathroom. However, if you don't, buy one at once, and make sure it is reliable and accurate. You may test the scale for accuracy by standing on it three times. If the readings are the same, the scale can be considered accurate. If you are an absolute stickler for perfection, you can get a guaranteed accurate scale from a medical supply house.

Place the scale in a convenient spot in your bathroom, and tape a chart on the wall directly above it, together with a pencil on a string so you won't fail to record your weight. At the same time, make a mental note that you will weigh yourself every day; in fact, you are going to weigh yourself every day for the rest of your life!

Your weight chart should be on a heavy piece of graph paper, which you can get at any stationery store. On the left hand side, starting at the top, list your present weight. Allowing one space on the graph paper for every pound, continue listing consecutive numbers from top to bottom. For example: your present weight (250) at the top left hand corner down to your desired weight (185) towards the bottom.

Along the bottom line, from left to right, insert the date, starting with the date you begin your program. Allow one space for each day.

You're now ready to begin charting your weight loss. In line with the first day's date, make a dot opposite your present weight figure at the top. This is your starting point, and being at the top of the chart, there is only one way to go—and that's down!

Each day you make another dot, indicating the day and the weight. After a week, you can start joining the dots, making a descending line indicating the progress you are making. People

SAMPLE WEIGHT CHART

WEIGHT

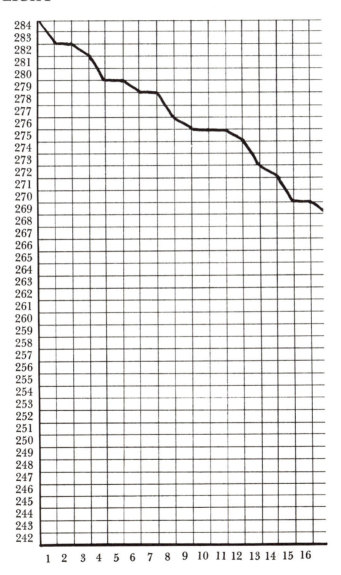

DAY & MONTH

tell me there is no greater thrill than watching that pencil line drop slowly down . . . and down . . . and down!

Do not become too disturbed if occasionally the line does not go down, but remains level or even goes up a bit. Many people (especially women) have fluid shift problems which make their weight loss line appear more like a stair step rather than a straight line. Remember all massive weight gains begin with the first five pounds, and it is far easier to restructure yourself and lose those five pounds than to wait until your obesity becomes totally out of hand.

When you have reached your desired weight level, there is a means to safeguard you from back-sliding, as can happen if you get careless. (Remember, psychostructure is a *permanent* means of weight control—provided you adhere to the program day in, day out, for the rest of your life).

Above your lowest weight level (your ultimate goal) draw a *yellow* pencil line four pounds above, and a *red* pencil line four pounds above the yellow line.

These are your danger signals. Continue recording your daily weight as usual, and if, for any reason, you find your weight increasing, the colored lines will serve as warning signals. If you reach the yellow line, it's time to start checking your diary to find out where you've been slipping! If you reach the red line, then it's crisis time, and you'd better do some serious thinking about your condition before it gets completely out of hand again. It is best at this time to reconsult your physician.

Does this mean that anyone losing weight through psychostructure *can* gain back all the weight that's lost? Of course you can—if you allow yourself to. Remember success depends on *you,* the patient, more than on *me, the doctor.* The system works, but only if you follow the rules.

The red and yellow lines on your weight chart serve as a reminder, plus a potential warning, to follow the daily routine in regard to diet, to exercise *and* to weighing yourself, all of which are essential contributions towards permanently ridding yourself of obesity. But the greatest danger lies in your *mind,* and its effect on your appetite.

We've discussed your daily diary and your weight chart.

Now let's discuss some of the ways you can guard yourself against unstructured eating, which is not only the prime cause of obesity, but is a constant threat to anyone on the psychostructure program.

All unstructured eating stems from some form of appetite stimulation, which is rarely spasmodic.

You are watching television at eleven o'clock at night. A food commercial comes on, and you watch it, aware that you had dinner four hours earlier. Maybe you see Mrs. Olsen extolling the virtues of mountain grown coffee, together with a plate of sweet rolls, or maybe a horde of precocious children are caterwauling over the joys of canned custard . . . whichever of the tempting assaults on our ears and eyes you happen to catch, it achieves the desired result: your mouth starts to water, you ease out of your chair, go to the kitchen, open the refrigerator and whammo! Ham . . . cheese . . . bread . . . mayonnaise . . . a dozen different temptations tantalize you in two seconds. By the time your program is back on the tube, you're back in your chair, munching an over-stuffed sandwich, and not feeling the slightest bit guilty over giving in to that irresistible compulsion.

The guilty party, of course, is the commercial, and because you were unable to structure your environment, and had not progressed sufficiently yet in restructuring your responses, you succumbed to the stimulation of the advertising. BUT . . . there is another factor to be considered. Your refrigerator. Admittedly it is impossible to eliminate TV commercials, but you can, and should, eliminate from easy reach any unstructured food in your kitchen. In your campaign against obesity, you must cover all fronts!

That brings us to some basic changes that I recommend very strongly to protect you against unstructured eating. Patients in my clinic do not have problems such as the above because they are in a controlled environment; but you, at home, are wide open to daily back-sliding unless you develop a number of restructured activities and routines connected with food.

First, you will most likely need to restructure your kitchen, which includes your pantry and freezer. This is part of the environmental control which is essential for the obesity-prone person in order to break a lifetime of bad habits. Environmental control means changing your environment so that it will help, not hinder, your effort to lose weight. This means turning a critical eye on the way food is kept in your kitchen. Do you keep a larder well-stocked in case of unexpected company? (That's *out*—if food is easily available to you at home, you're going to eat it!) Do you keep dishes of "snack-type" food around the house, such as nuts in the den, pretzels on top of the TV, candy by the telephone? (Food is to be kept in the kitchen *only*, and out of sight.) Go through your kitchen and pantry and eliminate all food that is not on your diet, and maintain only sufficient quantities of food for your weekly planned menu.

If you consider this impractical, consider the alternatives. There must be only food in your home that is on your diet, otherwise you're not going to succeed in losing weight. But what about when company arrives, you might say? Emergencies like this can be handled by a quick trip to the store. You must be more concerned with everyday eating than the unexpected drop-in guest. Plan your kitchen to suit *yourself*—and this means maintaining a food supply sufficient only for the weekly needs as prescribed in your diet. No party food or snack food. No calorie-laden concoctions for cocktail parties. Nothing, and I mean, *nothing* that is not on your list of approved food items.

Along with restructuring your kitchen, start the practice of planning your menu. Use your daily diary and a calorie guide, and write down your intended meals for the coming week. This enables you to make up your shopping list to include everything you need, and eliminate anything you *don't* need. Write your planned meals into your daily diary, sticking to the caloric limitations of your diet; then work out the quantities you will be required to purchase so that each meal will be complete, with *no leftovers*.

Some people go one step further, and group their shopping list into sections to match the location of food in their favorite supermarket. This means less time spent up and down the aisles, searching for food. Remember, the less time you spend at the market, the less likelihood there is for you to reach out for those items not on your list. In fact, the quicker you can get in and out of the market, the better. A supermarket is temptation with a capital T, so go there only when you have to, and always armed with your shopping list containing only those items you need, and in the quantities sufficient only for your weekly planned menu.

The calorie guide is a must in planning your menu, because there is no room for fudging when preparing your meals. You cannot throw in a little extra here and there, saying to yourself that it doesn't matter! *Every calorie counts!* Stick to your diet; stick to the ingredients listed, no more, no less! Many people have told me that their weekly planning sessions with menus and shopping lists are no longer a chore, but a pleasant new routine, when they realize how important this is in their overall program of losing weight.

Now let's talk about grocery shopping. Remember: the seeds of an episode of overeating are sown when you shop. Why do I say this? Because it's true! Even if you mentally vow that you're buying that ice cream for the rest of your family, it will still be a forbidden item in your freezer that, at some time or another, you'll find yourself consuming.

This is why your shopping list should be made out in advance, and should include only those items which you are allowed to eat. A good idea is to make up a "standard shopping list" containing *only* those items permitted in your diet; place a check mark against those things you intend buying, things you are needing, and *buy only those items,* and only in the quantities sufficient for your planned menu. Don't give in to temptation when you see something in the market that appeals to you, or which stimulates your appetite. As a double safeguard, always do your shopping as soon as possible after you have eaten. Try not to shop at eleven in the morning or at four in the afternoon, times when you normally start getting hungry. You must do everything possible to minimize your reaction to external stimuli, especially as you will be going into a veritable paradise of visual stimulation. (Those carefully laid-out displays in the market are traps for the unwary shopper whether he is overweight or not! Their purpose is to prompt you to buy, whether you need the item or not).

If you shop at a time when you feel the slightest bit hungry you'll find yourself weakening as you wander down the aisles, gazing at shelf after shelf of cookies, ice cream and delectable frozen temptations. So what happens? You load up your basket with items not on your list, items you shouldn't eat, and more importantly, items that have no business being inside your home. Even if your justify your actions by telling yourself that extra portion of food is for next week, it won't happen that way! You'll get home and gorge! Do I sound as though I have no faith in your adhering to your program? Right! I know from past experiences how easy it is to back-slide, which is why I stress, more than once in this book, that you must stick to the rules. And with shopping, the rules include going at a time when you are not hungry, using a preplanned list, and buying only those items on your list.

Always buy in controlled portions. Your diet menu may call for six ounces of steak, so ask the butcher to cut you a piece of steak *six ounces* in weight after the fat is all trimmed off. Don't buy twelve ounces and tell yourself you'll cut it in half when you get home. You won't! That twelve ounce piece will be under the broiler faster than you can blink your eyes! Buy only the amount of food called for in your diet.

This will naturally mean more frequent trips to the store, but the exercise will be good for you. In fact, if you live within walking distance of your local supermarket, you can combine your daily required walking with your needed shopping chores. Even better: walk to the store right after dinner. What better way to help your body burn up those calories you've eaten? And walking after dinner will eliminate the dangers of feeling hungry in the market and maybe succumbing to temptation.

Finally, avoid all convenience foods, which should be regarded as unstructured items in your diet. By convenience foods, I refer to such things as potato chips, cookies, pretzels, or prepackaged frozen dinners, that is, products that can be eaten merely by reaching for them, rather than those which require some preparation. You are far less likely to indulge in a plate of oatmeal, which takes time and effort to prepare, but you are liable to dig into a box of sugar snacks if it happens to be on the pantry shelf.

Some people will complain that such a strict regimen in regard to household food items is impossible, citing spouses and children as considerations that cannot be overlooked. Let me say that your going on a diet is not only for your own good, but also for your family as well. Certainly a husband should welcome a wife's efforts to lop off any excess flab. Any man feels happier and prouder of a slim, attractive mate than one who pants, puffs, and prowls the pantry at night instead of being in the bedroom!

Women also prefer their men slim and trim and loving rather than having a flabby, soft-toned man sitting in front of the TV with a double-decker sandwich. It is important to stress that men who live alone and do their own shopping and cooking should follow the same rules that are discussed here. Obese husbands should enlist the aid of their wives in trying to help them create the proper environment for their dieting success.

If your children complain because there is no ice cream in the freezer, send them down to the corner drugstore for a cone, and stress that they are to finish eating it before they return home. You *must* keep unstructured foods out of the house or suffer the consequences, and if your family cares about your planned weight reduction as much as you do, they shouldn't find an understocked larder too much of a hardship, especially when they realize you're serious about your diet program.

But, very importantly, by eliminating unstructured, garbage food from your kitchen and your home you are also helping your family. They too will learn to eat only when hungry and their own internal control mechanisms will be reinforced by the absence of temptation. As you benefit from your newly controlled home environment, your family will also be benefiting in a physically and psychologically positive way.

Strictly enforce these principles of food buying: shop only from a preplanned shopping list containing only items on your diet; shop only when you are not hungry, such as after you've had a meal; buy only specific portions; buy no convenience foods. These rules are essential for your maximum progress in losing weight. You may not consider them too significant, but believe me, they are. The secret of success in psychostructure is restructuring your lifestyle, which includes the way you purchase food. This rule, like every rule included in this book, is suggested for only one reason: to help you achieve your ultimate goal of a slender, healthy body. You've realized by now that to achieve this ambition, you may have to make some basic changes in your lifestyle. So what? I've had patients come into my office and say they'll do *anything* to lose weight. Changing your shopping habits is certainly not much to ask when you really think about it.

Now we come to the matter of food storage. In restructuring your environment, you'll be pounds ahead by storing food so that it cannot be conveniently reached or quickly prepared for consumption.

If items are able to be frozen, freeze them! Thawed, you might be tempted to nibble; but by the time you defrost and prepare something, your urge to eat will have diminished. Impulse eating can pass as quickly as it arises once the stimulation is removed.

If possible, place food in opaque containers, especially perishables in the refrigerator. If you can't see it, your appetite is less likely to be stimulated. Out of sight, out of mind . . . which is why you should use aluminum foil for wrapping food rather than plastic. Store only foods that need to be cooked before eating, and store only sufficient amounts to fulfill your weekly planned menu. Too much food in storage only increases the risk of your going on an eating binge, no matter if the items *are* frozen or take time to prepare. Finally, food must be stored where you cannot easily see it, such as on counter tops or tables. There should be no food in sight when you walk into your kitchen at any time other than during meal preparation.

Many people complain that this rule is impossible, that totally sanitizing the food environment is too much of an imposition on other members of the family who are not on a diet. Again, I say, this is a matter of family cooperation. During the initial period of weight loss, a dieter must usually adopt strict measures to guard against unstructured eating, and these actions must be understood by the rest of the family. A family conference can usually iron out any dissenting attitudes. By the time the new regimen has been established for a month or two, the old habit patterns have been broken, and the new kitchen routine becomes a matter of course for everyone. We are all creatures of habit, which is one of the basic reasons behind the unfortunate incidence of obesity in modern man—from childhood we get into the bad habit of overeating—and bad habits require strict methods of control.

Putting a lock on your food cupboards or pantry is another very effective way of guarding against unstructured eating. The time and trouble you take getting the key (hopefully hidden in an inaccessible spot!) will diminish your appetite urge, and often dispel it entirely. One patient of mine who locked up all the food in her kitchen (including a lock on the refrigerator) told me this system saved her two pounds of excess weight per week.

The actual preparation of food is a vital matter. Many people while cooking instinctively taste everything they prepare, and a taste turns into a mouthful, which leads inevitably to another mouthful, and another. . . . If you have to indulge in this practice, use only a small measuring spoon, or better still, wear a surgical mask while preparing food. Don't laugh! This is one sure way of preventing those instinctive and involuntary moments of food tasting. Remember that *every calorie counts.* (Chewing sugarless gum is another good way of preventing a stove-top tasting spree!)

Be extremely careful in the amount of food you prepare, cooking only sufficient for each meal, thereby avoiding leftovers. A small kitchen scale and measuring cups are essential in this respect. Remember that obese people have poor judgment in estimating food quantities, so don't trust yourself. Measure exactly down to the last ounce, and prepare your meals as quickly as possible; then leave the kitchen. The less time you spend in a food environment, the better off you are.

In preparing as well as serving, you should exercise portion control, and never serve family style. You know how many there will be for a meal, so measure your food accordingly, enough for each person, for each plate. No more. Avoid uneven portions of meat, for example, because if one piece is left over, someone is going to race through his meal to get it. (And that person could be *you!*)

The manner in which you prepare certain dishes can minimize or double the calorie count. Chicken, rolled in flour and fried, has twice the calories of chicken that is skinned and broiled. If you learn to look upon every item in your kitchen as a potential weight producer, you'll soon automatically guard against those extra little touches in preparing a dish that can add unnecessary calories.

Cooking fat is a well-known hazard for dieters, so I'll repeat what you probably already know: fry as few items as possible, but if you must, use a lecithin spray on your skillet which is not only non-stick, but non-caloric as well. Another alternative is to use a teflon pan with mineral oil, which is good for onions, mushrooms and even potatoes. Mineral oil is not unpleasant; it has no calories at all because it cannot be absorbed by the body. However, if you are taking vitamins, take them at least three hours before you eat anything fried in mineral oil. The absorption of certain vitamins is blocked by the presence of mineral oil in the gastrointestinal tract.

Even though fried foods should be kept to a minimum, anyone on a diet needs a little fat each day to enable the system to absorb needed vitamins, both natural and additive. You will notice in the sample diet which follows this chapter, I specify corn oil (liquid or margarine) which I consider best for cholesterol and triglyceride reasons.

Some revision in the way you serve your meals can be helpful in guarding against unstructured eating, which includes improper *amounts* as well as the wrong *type* of food.

Never serve family style, placing quantities of food on the table that would allow second and third helpings; prepare your meals in the kitchen, and prepare individual plates with controlled portions of each item.

Psychologically, it is beneficial if you use small plates rather than the usual large dinner plate. A six ounce steak on a large plate looks rather lost and lonely and creates the impression of a small meal; but on a small plate, a small portion of food looks larger, and your psychological satisfaction will be enhanced, which is a vitally important aspect in weight control.

As your system slowly adjusts to being satisfied with smaller portions, you will find yourself automatically eating less food; but this process is governed in large measure by your mental reactions—your psychostructure.

The *way* you eat is also very important. Your meals should

always be taken in the same place, a suitable specific area such as the dining room, so that when you sit down to a meal, food is all you are concentrating on. Make it a rule never to eat in the den, watching television, because eating then becomes secondary, or unconscious, and again, this tends to diminish your structured attitude towards your food, and can lead to loose eating habits.

I cannot stress too much the importance of having total control over the act of eating. Most obese people respond to their food environment in an unconscious manner. Studies have shown that if an overweight person is conscious of what he is eating, there is a tendency to eat less. A group of women were asked merely to record for one week what they ate, and every single woman in this group lost weight because they were conscious of what they were doing.

Just as your diet must be structured, so also must the act of eating become structured. After serving the food, you should wait at least one minute before starting to eat it. Families who say grace before meals are only helping the dieter, because the more leisurely a meal is consumed, the better it is, not only for the dieter, but for everyone.

Why?

Because waiting a minute, then taking a mouthful, putting down the knife and fork, chewing slowly, and savoring the taste of the food extends the time of the meal. Waiting a minute also tends to diffuse the reflex that many obese patients have, that almost instantaneous lunge for the plate, a voracious attack reminiscent of a hungry lion. These people do not attack their food; they eat it leisurely, a characteristic which obesity-prone patients must learn to cultivate. Exerting conscious control over the act of eating is essential, chewing slowly and extending the time of the meal.

You should try to take no less than twenty minutes to consume your food, because it takes about twenty minutes for the blood sugar to become high enough to give you the feeling of having had enough, a feeling of satiety as the dieticians call it. Wolfing down a plateful in five minutes may fill your stomach, but your brain is still sending out signals for more food; which leaves you with a feeling of wanting more that can result in an unstructured eating episode later.

75

Eating slowly also tends to provide a deeper psychological satisfaction. Obese people who eat too quickly usually finish their meal before others at the table, making them feel that they have been deprived. This can lead to wanting (and sometimes getting) second helpings which, of course, can be disastrous in a structured eating program.

After a meal, if there are any leftovers unless they have previously been assigned to use at a subsequent specific meal these should be discarded in such a way no one will be able to retrieve them. The trash can is not good enough; I have known some patients who've admitted raiding the trash after a meal, searching desperately and uncontrollably for that extra smidgen of food! If you have one, use the disposal or trash compactor, incinerator, or outside garbage can.

Get rid of leftovers at once if you're serious about getting rid of your overweight. If this offends your sense of economy, let me remind you that the cost of leftover food is negligible compared with the cost of having medical help for your obesity.

After the meal, leave the table at once. If you must continue sitting over coffee, make sure any remaining food is removed from sight. After a half-hour's chit-chat, you can easily pick at morsels left on someone's plate, thereby succumbing to unstructured eating and adding unwanted calories to your system.

That's it! That's how psychostructure works, but in addition to changing many of your daily habits and altering your lifestyle, you have to limit your food intake—go on a diet. The following chapter lists not only recipes for my prescribed diet, but a daily menu for four weeks, plus many other taste-tempting recipes that do not exceed your caloric limitations.

Initially, you will be restricted to 700 calories a day, which has proven to be ideal. The reason being that at the 700 calorie level, there is sufficient leeway to include those items in the diet which I consider essential. Diets containing more than 700 calories per day merely slow down the process of weight loss. I can speak from personal experience that the feelings of hunger are no different at 700 calories than they are at 1100 or 1200 calories. Nothing is more discouraging than to stay on a diet with an extremely small weight loss, even though eventually a normal, ideal weight may be achieved.

However, once you have achieved your desired weight level, you may increase your daily calorie intake, but only as follows: after reaching your ideal weight, increase your daily calories by 200. If you continue, by the end of that week, to lose weight, increase them by another 200. Continue to increase your calorie intake by 200 per day until you find that you are neither losing nor gaining. At that point, you will have reached your particular individual maintenance calorie allotment. Ingesting this number of calories will thereafter keep your weight constant.

Of course, changes in lifestyle, increase in exercise, decrease in activity, etc., may change this, so you will have to monitor your weight carefully each day and continue making whatever adjustments in calories may be necessary.

Some patients have been able to maintain their desired weight with as many as 2500 calories a day *after* completing their initial weight loss; but this is something you can only determine with time. But you *must always* start your diet at 700 calories a day. In general, most women can maintain their ideal weight on 1500 calories daily, while many men tend to balance out around 2500 per day.

Often I am asked, "May I skip breakfast and lunch and have a larger meal at night?" The answer is *no*. To become successful in achieving normal weight, an obese person *must eat three meals a day*. Each meal should contain the prescribed number of calories, or less, but if you do save 100 calories at lunch, you may not add these on to dinner. Why? Because this practice tends to get people into the habit of eating larger and larger meals at night; then they will add in breakfast and lunch, and before you know it, the daily calories are skyrocketing. Stick to my daily menu as outlined in the following chapter. There is an appealing variety of dishes, plus many extra recipes; however, should you desire an even wider variety, you may substitute, provided your substitution does not exceed the number of calories specified for each meal.

You will notice, in general, breakfast and lunch contain 150 calories each; dinner around 400. But, for example, should you prefer *Product 19* cereal to the puffed wheat and puffed rice listed, go ahead, but realize that *Product 19* has six calories more per serving than puffed wheat or rice; so use proportionately less skim milk to keep your total calories at 150 for that meal.

Remember it's the calories that count, and your daily diary will tell you whether or not you are keeping your diet within limits.

Remember the Fifth Commandment of Psychostructure: *To control what I eat, I must control my environment.*

6. YOUR NEW DAILY DIET

Before listing your daily diet, I am giving you the recipes for many of the items included in the daily food allotment. Not only will you find these recipes delicious, but they are very economical, certainly something to be welcomed with today's rising prices. More important, they are economical in calories, which is the most important aspect of all! For example, twelve ounces of my vegetable soup with one and a half ounces of chicken total approximately 150 calories—considerably less than the canned soup you buy in the market, and at about half the price.

Many of these items can be prepared ahead of time and kept frozen, which is not only an added convenience but again a savings in time and effort. I suggest you set a certain day on which to start your diet, and give yourself a few days beforehand in which to prepare and freeze many of the recipes which follow.

In recipes that call for artificial sweetener, one package is equal to the sweetness of two teaspoons of sugar.

VEGETABLE SOUP

My vegetable soup can be prepared from either beef stock or chicken stock, giving you a variety of flavor. Serving portions of soup, plus beef or chicken, can be frozen and then merely defrosted and heated prior to your meal.

BEEF STOCK

You will need a gallon (or about 16 cups) of water and a large pot. Bring the water to a boil and add beef and beef bones. A pound to a pound and a half is sufficient. Reduce the heat and simmer for one hour. Remove the meat and the bones, reserving the cooked meat. Strain the liquid into another pot and place in the refrigerator overnight. The next day remove all the solidified fat from the top of the stock.

CHICKEN STOCK

Prepare the same as for beef stock, substituting a small chicken fryer (approximately a pound and a half to two pounds), cut up, instead of the beef. To insure the chicken is completely covered during the cooking, I suggest you cut the chicken into small pieces. Remove the chicken pieces and set aside to cool. Strain the liquid into another pot and place in refrigerator overnight. The next day remove all the solidified fat from the top of the stock. Meanwhile, when cool, remove the meat from the chicken bones, discarding all skin and bones, and reserving the meat for later use.

TO PREPARE THE SOUP

You will need:

2 cups of diced celery
2 cups of diced onions
2 cups of diced carrots

4 cups of diced tomatoes
2 cups of chopped cabbage
1 small can (6 oz.) of tomato paste

Add the vegetables and the tomato paste to either your chicken or beef stock, season with your favorite spices and simmer at low heat for thirty minutes.

Divide into serving portions of twelve ounces each, adding to the beef stock, one ounce of the reserved cooked beef; and to the chicken stock, one and a half ounces of the reserved cooked chicken. Place the portions in plastic containers and store in the freezer until needed, at which time you merely place the plastic container in a pot of boiling water for twenty minutes, or until defrosted and hot.

For seafood fans, you may vary this recipe and make clam chowder and crab gumbo by substituting clams and crabmeat for the beef, as follows:

CLAM CHOWDER

For a serving of 133 calories, add one half cup of cooked clams (78 calories) to eight ounces of the beef stock vegetable soup (55 calories), season with thyme and serve hot. Delicious!

CRAB GUMBO

For a serving of 157 calories, add three ounces of cooked crabmeat (85 calories), one-quarter cup cooked okra (17 calories) to eight ounces of the beef stock vegetable soup (55 calories), season to taste and serve hot. Out of this world!

Another tempting variation for soup fans is the following:

SPINACH SOUP

You will need:

2 cups of chicken broth
1 tbsp. corn oil margarine
1 clove of garlic, coarsely
   chopped

1 minced scallion (or
   very small onion)
1 pkg. frozen chopped
   spinach (10 ounces)

Melt the margarine in a saucepan over a low flame. Do not let it brown. Add the garlic and cook for two minutes over low heat. Add the scallion and simmer for five minutes or until transparent. Add the chicken broth and the spinach and allow to simmer at a slow gentle boil until the spinach is defrosted (about ten minutes). Serve piping hot with a generous pinch of chopped fresh parsley sprinkled over the top. Serving portions are the same as for beef or chicken soup, twelve ounces each.

We'll move on now to my salad recipes, which are a frequent and important part of my diet—all low calorie, and all easy to prepare and very tasty.

CUCUMBER SALAD

Slice one large cucumber (29 calories) either with or without the skin and sprinkle with one quarter of a medium onion, finely chopped (10 calories). Cover with vinegar dressing (see page 84) which has no calories. Makes one portion. Total calories: 39.

BEET SALAD

Slice one half cup cooked beets (25 calories), sprinkle with one quarter of a medium onion, finely chopped (10 calories). Cover with vinegar dressing (see page 84). Makes one portion. Total calories: 35.

GREEN BEAN SALAD

Sprinkle one quarter of a medium onion, finely chopped (10 calories) over one half cup cooked string beans (15 calories). Add enough vinegar dressing to coat the beans. Makes one portion. Total calories: 25.

DIET COLE SALAD

Prepare a bowl of this salad and keep it covered in the refrigerator, adding the dressing only at the time of serving.

Shred one small fresh cabbage, two carrots, and one green pepper. Combine and stir briskly to insure even distribution of the carrot and pepper. Before serving, add vinegar dressing to coat the ingredients. Total calories per half-cup portion: 15.

SPINACH SALAD

Coarsely chop up half a cup of raw, fresh spinach (20 calories). Add one chopped, cooked egg white (15 calories) and one ounce of diet French dressing (30 calories). Toss lightly and serve. Makes one portion. Total calories: 65.

BEET AND COTTAGE CHEESE SALAD

You will need:

1 cup cooked chopped beets	1½ cups water
1 cup cottage cheese	2 pkgs. of artificial sweetner
1 envelope unflavored gelatin	¼ cup fresh lemon juice

Over a low flame, place one envelope of unflavored gelatin (28 calories) in a saucepan with one half cup of water. Add artificial sweetner (3 calories) and stir until dissolved. Remove from stove and add one cup water and one quarter cup lemon juice (24 calories). Chill in the refrigerator until the mixture begins to jell (about the consistency of unbeaten egg whites). Stir in one cup of cooked, chopped beets (50 calories) and one cup of cottage cheese (200 calories). Divide equally into six individual dessert cups and replace in refrigerator and allow to set thoroughly. One serving: 50 calories.

PERFECTION SALAD

You will need:

½ cup shredded cabbage
1 cup chopped celery
½ medium sized red pepper, chopped
½ medium sized green pepper, chopped

1 envelope unflavored gelatin
1½ cups water
1 pkg. of artificial sweetener
1 tbsp. fresh lemon juice

Over a low flame, place one envelope of unflavored gelatin (28 calories) in a saucepan with one half cup of water, add artificial sweetener (one and a half calories) and stir until dissolved. Remove from stove and add one cup water and one tablespoon of lemon juice (4 calories). Chill in the refrigerator until the mixture begins to jell (about the consistency of unbeaten egg whites).

Stir in one half cup shredded cabbage (15 calories), one cup chopped celery (20 calories), one half medium sized red pepper, chopped (8 calories) and one half medium sized green pepper, chopped (10 calories). Divide into four individual dessert cups and replace in refrigerator and allow to set thoroughly. One serving: 22 calories.

VINEGAR DRESSING

Fill a pint jar with one and a half cups of vinegar. Add one half cup of water and one and one half packages of artificial sweetener. Shake well, and store in the refrigerator for use when needed. This dressing contains virtually no calories.

For some meat and fish recipes in the diet, tomato sauce is mentioned. The following recipe should be used to prepare the tomato sauce, which can be frozen and used as needed. You may store the sauce in one cup portions, or in an ice cube tray. One frozen cube equals one ounce, or twelve calories.

BASIC TOMATO SAUCE

You will need:

6-8 medium tomatoes,
  preferably vine-ripened for
  flavor and rich color
1 large onion, finely diced
1 large green pepper,
  finely diced

3-4 cloves of garlic,
  coarsely chopped
1 tsp. black pepper
1 tsp. oregano, if desired
1 tsp. sweet basil, if desired
artificial sweetener, to taste
1 cup of basic beef stock

Simmer all the ingredients together over a low flame until the vegetables are soft and the mixture begins to thicken. Add extra beef broth if necessary to make four cups. As with any sauce, the flavor is enhanced by lengthy *slow* cooking. Do not allow the mixture to come to a rolling boil at any time. Puree into a smooth sauce either by repeated straining or in a blender.

Allow to cool and freeze. A two ounce portion has 25 calories.

Who said you had to give up baked potatoes? These are included in my diet, deliciously stuffed as follows:

STUFFED BAKED POTATO

You will need:

1/2 baked potato
1/4 cup cottage cheese

Chives

Scoop the potato out of the skin and mash with the cottage cheese and chives. Replace in the skin and pop back in a 400 degree oven to lightly brown the top. Makes one serving. Total calories: 100.

Another mouth-watering taste treat is Shrimp Creole, usually regarded as a weight producing gourmet meal—but not the way the following recipe is prepared.

SHRIMP CREOLE

You will need:

1 can unsweetened tomatoes	1 pkg. of artificial sweetener
2 medium green peppers	1 tsp. chili powder
1 medium-size onion	1 clove garlic or
½ cup chopped celery	garlic powder
20 oz. fresh shrimp	1 bay leaf

Combine in a large sauce pan all the ingredients and simmer gently for thirty minutes. Add a dash of Tabasco and salt substitute to taste. Again, cook gently and do not allow to come to a rolling boil. This recipe makes four servings with a total of 840 calories. To serve, place one portion (210 calories) over a half cup of cooked rice (100 calories). Wickedly delicious!

The next recipe proves that gourmet meals are not *verboten* to dieters. I'm sure even Julia Child would approve the following recipe for *Coq Au Vin,* or Chicken in Burgundy, which you could serve for a special dinner for guests who would never realize they were eating a low-calorie meal!

COQ AU VIN

You will need:

3 whole boned medium sized chicken breasts (with skin removed)	1 tsp. marjoram
	1 tsp. thyme
	2 tbsp. chopped parsley
1 tbsp. corn oil margarine	12 small, white boiling
1 cup of beef stock	onions, peeled
½ cup burgundy wine	4 stalks of celery, whole

Cut the chicken breasts in half and brown in a large skillet in the corn oil margarine, about five to seven minutes. Add: the beef stock, wine, thyme, marjoram, parsley and onions. Cover with celery stalks and cook slowly for one hour over low heat with the lid tightly on the skillet. To serve, discard the celery stalks, remove the chicken and onions to a platter and spoon over the gravy, which you may have to simmer a while longer until it is reduced and thickened. Total servings: 6. Total calories per serving: 187.

Many dieters regard omelets as being beyond their caloric limitations. Not if you stick to the following recipe.

EGG-VEGETABLE OMELET

You will need:

3 egg whites
½ medium sized onion, chopped
½ medium sized green pepper, chopped

½ cup mushrooms, sliced
¼ cup cottage cheese
½ tbsp. corn oil margarine
½ cup diet tomato sauce, heated

Whip three egg whites (45 calories) until fluffy, but not dry. Fold in: one half chopped onion (20 calories), one half chopped green pepper (10 calories), one half cup mushrooms (20 calories), one quarter cup cottage cheese (50 calories). Cook in a large skillet greased with ½ tbsp. of corn oil margarine, using a low flame. When the bottom is slightly brown, flip over and cover with a lid for a few minutes until cooked. Serve topped with one half cup of diet tomato sauce (see page 85), hot. Total number of calories: 245. Amount of eating enjoyment: unlimited!

Here comes a gourmet recipe again. (No wonder so many of my patients can hardly believe they're on a diet!)

SCALLOPS IN WHITE WINE

You will need:

1¼ lbs. scallops
1 cup dry white wine
4 small white onions, chopped

1 clove garlic, minced
1 tsp. fresh parsley, chopped
black pepper to taste

Pre-heat the oven to 400 degrees.
Place the scallops in a baking dish and cover with one cup of

dry white wine. Cover with four small chopped white onions and one minced clove of garlic. Sprinkle with black pepper and a teaspoon of chopped parsley. Bake for ten minutes, or until the scallops are done. Weigh six ounces *after cooking* (scallops shrink during cooking) and serve garnished with lemon slices and paprika. Total calories per six ounce serving: 240.

Now we come to casseroles, always a favorite at mealtimes, especially in the winter.

SPINACH CASSEROLE

You will need:

1 cup spinach, cooked, chopped and well-drained	¼ medium sized tomato, thinly sliced
½ cup cottage cheese	

Mix thoroughly one cup of cooked, chopped spinach, well drained (40 calories), together with one half cup of cottage cheese (100 calories). Bake in a 375 degree oven until the mixture is hot and bubbling. Remove and serve, topped with one quarter medium sized tomato thinly sliced (10 calories). Makes one portion. Total calories: 150.

EGGPLANT CASSEROLE

You will need:

1 cup eggplant, boiled and diced	¼ medium sized tomato, thinly sliced
¼ cup cottage cheese	oregano to taste
½ cup diet tomato sauce	garlic powder to taste

Stir together thoroughly: one cup of diced, boiled eggplant (40 calories), one quarter cup cottage cheese (50 calories). Place in a casserole, pour one half cup of diet tomato sauce (see page 85) (50 calories) over the top and sprinkle with oregano and garlic powder to taste. Bake in a 375 degree oven until the mixture is hot and bubbling. Remove and serve, topped with thinly sliced tomato (10 calories). Makes one portion. Total calories: 150.

TUNA CASSEROLE

You will need:

3 oz. tuna (packed in water)
well-drained
¾ cup cottage cheese

1 tbsp. onion chopped
1 tbsp. green pepper
chopped

Mix tuna with cottage cheese, onion and green pepper. Add pepper and spices to taste. Place the mixture in a casserole and bake in a 350 degree oven for thirty minutes. Remove and place under the broiler briefly to brown the top. Serve garnished with lemon wedges and parsley. Makes one serving. Total calories: 310.

BAKED APPLE

You will need:

4 medium sized apples
1 can diet lemon soda

cinnamon to taste
Artificial sweetener

Core the apples, leaving the skins on. Place in a baking dish and sprinkle with cinammon and artificial sweetener. Pour one can of Diet Lemon Soda over the apples and bake in a 350 degree oven for forty-five minutes or until the apples are fork soft. Total calories in half a baked apple: 40.

Now that the recipes have whetted your curiosity and shown that diet meals need not be either monotonous or uninspired, you are ready to see how they fill out the daily diet, which you have divided into four weeks. After completing your fourth week, you simply go back to the plan for week one and begin the cycle again. You may make substitutions where indicated, but remember to keep track of everything you eat in your diary, and count your calories!

In cooking vegetables, I would suggest that steaming is preferable to boiling. Do yourself a nutritional favor and buy a steamer, if you don't already have one. And remember that vegetables are better crispy and slightly under-cooked than overcooked to a pulp.

FIRST WEEK
MONDAY

BREAKFAST: *Calories*

4 oz. orange juice	55
1 serving of puffed wheat or puffed rice	55
½ cup of skim milk	45
TOTAL:	155

LUNCH:

Spinach casserole	150
One fourth of a tomato	10
TOTAL:	160

DINNER:

6 oz. broiled chicken	300
with 2 tbsp. diet tomato sauce	25
½ cup carrots (boiled)	20
½ cup broccoli (boiled)	20
Small tossed salad	10
with 1 oz. diet dressing	30
TOTAL:	405

TOTAL CALORIES FOR THIS DAY: 720

If preferred, or for variety, you may substitute a 5 oz. beef patty (broiled) instead of chicken.

FIRST WEEK
TUESDAY

BREAKFAST: *Calories*

½ grapefruit   50
1 serving of puffed wheat or puffed rice   55
½ cup of skim milk   45

TOTAL: 150

LUNCH:

Fruit plate, consisting of:
½ cup diet pineapple   40
¼ cup diet cherries   20
¼ cup diet blueberries   20
¼ cup diet peaches   20
¼ cup cottage cheese   50

TOTAL: 150

DINNER:

5 oz. shrimp creole   210
½ cup rice   100
½ cup green beans   15
½ cup summer squash   15
Small tossed salad   10
with 1 oz. diet dressing   30
15 grapes   30

TOTAL: 410

TOTAL CALORIES FOR THIS DAY: 710

If desired, or for variety, you may substitute 5 oz. of broiled
chicken instead of shrimp.

FIRST WEEK
WEDNESDAY

BREAKFAST: *Calories*

½ baked apple 40
½ cup oatmeal 65
with ½ cup of skim milk 45

TOTAL: 150

LUNCH:

2 oz. tuna (packed in water) 100
on a large lettuce salad 20
with 1 oz. diet dressing 30

TOTAL: 150

DINNER:

4 oz. broiled beef liver 240
with 1 medium broiled onion 40
½ baked potato 50
¼ acorn squash 35
Apple gelatin salad 30

TOTAL: 395

TOTAL CALORIES FOR THIS DAY: 695

If desired, or for variety, you may substitute 5 oz. of broiled chicken instead of liver.

FIRST WEEK
THURSDAY

BREAKFAST: *Calories*

½ banana   45
1 serving of puffed wheat or puffed rice   55
with ½ cup of skim milk   45

TOTAL: 145

LUNCH:

3 oz. cooked shrimp with celery   100
1 medium tomato   35
1 oz. diet cocktail sauce   15

TOTAL: 150

DINNER:

6 oz. broiled flounder   290
½ cup stewed tomatoes   25
6 asparagus spears   20
½ cup diet cole slaw   15
1 tangerine   40

TOTAL: 390

TOTAL CALORIES FOR THIS DAY: 685

If desired, or for variety, you may substitute a 5 oz. broiled beef
patty instead of flounder.

FIRST WEEK
FRIDAY

BREAKFAST: *Calories*

½ cup citrus sections   55
½ cup of Cream of Wheat   50
with ½ cup of skim milk   45

TOTAL: 150

LUNCH:

Hot vegetable plate, including:
½ cup broccoli   20
½ cup squash   15
½ cup beets   30
¼ cup cottage cheese   50
with 1 oz. diet dressing   30

TOTAL: 145

DINNER:

5 oz. steak (broiled)   300
½ baked potato   50
Large tossed salad   20
with 1 oz. diet dressing   30

TOTAL: 400

TOTAL CALORIES FOR THIS DAY: 695

If desired, or for variety, you may substitute 6 oz. of broiled
chicken instead of the steak.

FIRST WEEK
SATURDAY

BREAKFAST: *Calories*

½ cup diet cherries   40
½ cup cottage cheese   100

TOTAL: 140

LUNCH:

2 oz. tuna (packed in water)   100
Large lettuce salad   20
with 1 oz. diet dressing   30

TOTAL: 150

DINNER:

6 oz. broiled chicken   300
½ cup carrots   20
½ cup cauliflower   10
One-eighth helping diet apple pie   56

TOTAL: 386

TOTAL CALORIES FOR THIS DAY: 676

If desired, or for variety, you may substitute a 5 oz. broiled beef patty instead of chicken.

FIRST WEEK
SUNDAY

BREAKFAST: *Calories*

½ grapefruit	50
1 helping of puffed wheat or puffed rice	55
with ½ cup of skim milk	45
TOTAL:	150

LUNCH:

Beef vegetable soup:

12 oz. vegetable soup with 1 oz. beef	140
TOTAL:	140

DINNER:

Tuna casserole	310
6 asparagus spears	20
Salad, consisting of:	
½ cucumber	15
½ tomato	20
¼ onion	10
in lettuce leaves with vinegar dressing	5
½ peach	20
TOTAL:	400

TOTAL CALORIES FOR THIS DAY: 690

If desired, or for variety, you may substitute a 5 oz. broiled beef patty instead of tuna.

For those of you who prefer to sleep late and skip breakfast on Sundays, the following brunch menu may be substituted for breakfast *and* lunch:

SUNDAY BRUNCH: *Calories*

½ grapefruit 50
Egg-Vegetable Omelet 245
TOTAL: 295

SECOND WEEK
MONDAY

BREAKFAST: *Calories*

½ orange   40
1 helping of puffed wheat or puffed rice   55
with ½ cup of skim milk   45

                              TOTAL: 140

LUNCH:

8 oz. vegetable soup   55
with 2 tbsp. barley   34
and 1 oz. of beef   60

                              TOTAL: 149

DINNER:

5 oz. broiled beef patty   300
½ cup green beans   15
½ cup beets   30
Large tossed salad   20
with 1 oz. diet dressing   30

                              TOTAL: 395

TOTAL CALORIES FOR THIS DAY: 684

If desired, or for variety, you may substitute 6 oz. broiled chicken
instead of the beef patty.

SECOND WEEK
TUESDAY

BREAKFAST: *Calories*

½ baked apple	40
½ cup oatmeal	65
with ½ cup of skim milk	45
TOTAL:	150

LUNCH:

Spinach casserole	150
TOTAL:	150

DINNER:

6 oz. broiled flounder	290
½ cup broccoli	20
½ acorn squash	35
½ grapefruit	50
TOTAL:	395

TOTAL CALORIES FOR THIS DAY: 695

If desired, or for variety, you may substitute 5 oz. broiled beef patty for the flounder.

SECOND WEEK
WEDNESDAY

BREAKFAST: *Calories*

4 oz. orange juice	55
1 serving of puffed wheat or puffed rice	55
with ½ cup of skim milk	45
TOTAL:	155

LUNCH:

2 oz. tuna (packed in water)	100
Large lettuce salad	20
with 1 oz. diet dressing	30
TOTAL:	150

DINNER:

4 oz. roast beef	240
½ stuffed baked potato	100
½ cup cooked cabbage	20
½ cup beet & onion salad	35
TOTAL:	395

TOTAL CALORIES FOR THIS DAY 700

If desired, or for variety, you may substitute 5 oz. broiled chicken instead of the roast beef.

SECOND WEEK
THURSDAY

BREAKFAST: *Calories*

¾ cup strawberries   45
½ cup cottage cheese   100

                              TOTAL: 145

LUNCH:

2 oz. white turkey meat   100
¼ tomato   10
⅛ head lettuce   10
with 1 oz. diet dressing   30

                              TOTAL: 150

DINNER:

6 oz. scallops in wine   240
½ cup chopped spinach   20
1 broiled tomato   35
½ cup diet cole slaw   15
1 baked apple   80

                              TOTAL: 390

TOTAL CALORIES FOR THIS DAY: 685

If desired, or for variety, you may substitute 5 oz. broiled chicken
instead of the scallops.

SECOND WEEK
FRIDAY

BREAKFAST: *Calories*

1 tangerine	40
1 serving of puffed wheat or puffed rice	55
with ½ cup of skim milk	45
TOTAL:	140

LUNCH:

3 oz. cooked shrimp & celery	100
with 1 oz. diet cocktail sauce	15
½ tomato	20
Vegetable strips, as follows:	
2 celery, 2 green pepper, 2 carrot	15
TOTAL:	150

DINNER:

5 oz. broiled steak	300
½ cup carrots	20
½ cup brussels sprouts	20
½ cup green bean & onion salad	20
20 grapes	40
TOTAL:	400

TOTAL CALORIES FOR THIS DAY: 690

If desired, or for variety, you may substitute 6 oz. broiled chicken instead of the steak.

SECOND WEEK
SATURDAY

BREAKFAST: *Calories*

1 apple	75
1 orange	75
TOTAL:	150

LUNCH:

3 oz. salmon (packed in water)	120
1 tbsp. onion	5
¼ tomato	10
Small lettuce salad	10
TOTAL:	145

DINNER:

6 oz. broiled chicken	300
2 tbsp. tomato sauce	25
½ cup broccoli	20
½ cup beets	30
½ diet peach	20
TOTAL:	395

TOTAL CALORIES FOR THIS DAY: 690

If desired, or for variety, you may substitute a 5 oz. broiled beef patty instead of chicken.

SECOND WEEK
SUNDAY

BREAKFAST: *Calories*

4 oz. orange juice   55
1 serving of puffed wheat or puffed rice   55
with ½ cup of skim milk   45

TOTAL: 155

LUNCH:

12 oz. vegetable soup with 1 oz. beef   140

TOTAL: 140

DINNER:

5 oz. broiled beef patty   300
½ baked potato   50
Large tossed salad   20
with 1 oz. diet dressing   30

TOTAL: 400

TOTAL CALORIES FOR THIS DAY: 695

If you desire, or for variety, you may substitute 6 oz. broiled
chicken instead of the beef patty.

For those of you who prefer to sleep late and skip breakfast on Sundays, the following brunch menu may be substituted for breakfast *and* lunch:

SUNDAY BRUNCH: *Calories*

½ cup fresh orange juice 55
Egg-Vegetable Omelet 245

TOTAL: 300

THIRD WEEK
MONDAY

BREAKFAST: *Calories*

½ banana 45
1 serving of puffed wheat or puffed rice 55
with ½ cup of skim milk 45

　　　　　　　　　TOTAL: 145

LUNCH:

Diet fruit plate:
½ cup pineapple chunks 40
¼ cup cherries 20
¼ cup blueberries 20
¼ cup peaches 20
¼ cup cottage cheese 50

　　　　　　　　　TOTAL: 150

DINNER:

5 oz. shrimp creole 210
½ cup rice 100
6 asparagus spears 20
½ cup diet cole slaw 15
½ cup pineapple chunks 40

　　　　　　　　　TOTAL: 385

TOTAL CALORIES FOR THIS DAY: 680

If desired, or for variety, you may substitute a 5 oz. broiled beef patty (without rice) instead of the shrimp.

THIRD WEEK
TUESDAY

BREAKFAST: *Calories*

½ grapefruit   50
1 serving of puffed wheat or puffed rice   55
with ½ cup of skim milk   45

                         TOTAL: 150

LUNCH:

Clam chowder:
8 oz. beef stock soup   55
½ cup cooked clams   78

                         TOTAL: 133

DINNER:

5 oz. roast beef   300
½ baked potato   50
½ cup green beans   15
Apple salad   30

                         TOTAL: 395

TOTAL CALORIES FOR THIS DAY: 678

If desired, or for variety, you may substitute 6 oz. of broiled chicken
instead of the roast beef.

THIRD WEEK
WEDNESDAY

BREAKFAST: *Calories*

½ baked apple 40
½ cup oatmeal 65
with ½ cup of skim milk 45

TOTAL: 150

LUNCH:

Hot Vegetable Plate:
½ cup broccoli 20
½ cup summer squash 15
½ cup beets 30
¼ cup cottage cheese 50
with 1 oz. diet dressing 30

TOTAL: 145

DINNER:

6 oz. baked chicken 300
2 tbsp. tomato sauce 25
½ cup carrots with dill 20
½ cup brussels sprouts 20
Small lettuce salad 10
with 1 oz. diet dressing 30

TOTAL: 405

TOTAL CALORIES FOR THIS DAY: 700

If desired, or for variety, you may substitute a 5 oz. broiled beef patty for the chicken.

THIRD WEEK
THURSDAY

BREAKFAST: *Calories*

½ cup diet cherries   40
½ cup cottage cheese   100

TOTAL: 140

LUNCH:

2 oz. tuna (packed in water)   100
¼ tomato   10
Small lettuce salad   10
with 1 oz. diet dressing   30

TOTAL: 150

DINNER:

Tuna casserole   310
½ cup spinach   20
1 broiled tomato   35
½ cup diet cole slaw   15
½ diet peach   20

TOTAL: 400

TOTAL CALORIES FOR THIS DAY: 690

If desired, or for variety, you may substitute a 5 oz. broiled beef patty instead of tuna.

THIRD WEEK
FRIDAY

BREAKFAST: *Calories*

4 oz. orange juice	55
1 serving of puffed wheat or puffed rice	55
with 4 oz. of skim milk	45
TOTAL:	155

LUNCH:

Spinach casserole	150
TOTAL:	150

DINNER:

5 oz. broiled steak	300
½ baked potato	50
Large tossed salad	20
with 1 oz. diet dressing	30
TOTAL:	400

TOTAL CALORIES FOR THIS DAY: 705

If desired, or for variety, you may substitute 6 oz. broiled chicken instead of the steak.

THIRD WEEK
SATURDAY

BREAKFAST: *Calories*

1 tangerine   40
1 serving of puffed wheat or puffed rice   55
with 4 oz. of skim milk   45

TOTAL: 140

LUNCH:

2 oz. turkey   100
⅛ head lettuce   10
¼ tomato   10
with 1 oz. diet dressing   30

TOTAL: 150

DINNER:

5 oz. beef patty   300
½ cup carrots   20
½ cup green beans   15
½ cup: beet & onion salad   35
½ cup strawberries   30

TOTAL: 400

TOTAL CALORIES FOR THIS DAY: 690

If desired, or for variety, you may substitute 6 oz. broiled chicken
instead of the beef patty.

THIRD WEEK
SUNDAY

BREAKFAST: *Calories*

½ grapefruit   50
1 serving of puffed wheat or puffed rice   55
with ½ cup of skim milk   45

TOTAL: 150

LUNCH:

12 oz. vegetable beef soup with 1 oz. beef   140

TOTAL: 140

DINNER:

6 oz. broiled chicken   300
6 asparagus spears   20
½ cup mashed rutabagas   43
Large tossed salad   20
with 1 oz. diet dressing   30

TOTAL: 413

TOTAL CALORIES FOR THIS DAY: 703

If desired, or for variety, you may substitute 5 oz. broiled beef patty
for the chicken.

For those of you who prefer to sleep late and skip breakfast on Sundays, the following brunch menu may be substituted for breakfast *and* lunch:

SUNDAY BRUNCH: *Calories*

½ grapefruit   50
Egg-Vegetable Omelet   245
TOTAL: 295

FOURTH WEEK
MONDAY

BREAKFAST: *Calories*

½ cup citrus sections   55
½ cup cottage cheese   100

TOTAL: 155

LUNCH:

2 oz. tuna (packed in water)   100
¼ tomato   10
⅛ head lettuce   10
with 1 oz. diet dressing   30

TOTAL: 150

DINNER:

4 oz. roast beef   240
½ baked potato   50
½ cup green beans   15
Large lettuce salad   20
with 1 oz. diet dressing   30
½ orange   40

TOTAL: 395

TOTAL CALORIES FOR THIS DAY: 700

If desired, or for variety, you may substitute 6 oz. broiled chicken instead of the roast beef.

FOURTH WEEK
TUESDAY

BREAKFAST: *Calories*

25 grapes	50
1 serving of puffed wheat or puffed rice	55
with ½ cup of skim milk	45
TOTAL:	150

LUNCH:

2 oz. turkey	100
¼ tomato	10
⅛ head lettuce	10
with 1 oz. diet dressing	30
TOTAL:	150

DINNER:

6 oz. broiled flounder	290
½ cup zucchini squash with tomatoes	20
½ cup carrots	20
½ cup diet cole slaw	15
¾ cup fresh strawberries	45
TOTAL:	390

TOTAL CALORIES FOR THIS DAY: 690

If desired, or for variety, you may substitute a 5 oz. broiled beef patty for the flounder.

115

FOURTH WEEK
WEDNESDAY

BREAKFAST: *Calories*

½ baked apple   40
½ cup oatmeal   65
with ½ cup of skim milk   45

                      TOTAL: 150

LUNCH:

Spinach casserole   150

                      TOTAL: 150

DINNER:

6 oz. broiled chicken   300
2 tbsp. tomato sauce   25
½ cup broccoli   20
½ cup summer squash   15
1 tangerine   40

                      TOTAL: 400

TOTAL CALORIES FOR THIS DAY: 700

If desired, or for variety, you may substitute a 5 oz. broiled beef
patty for the chicken.

FOURTH WEEK
THURSDAY

BREAKFAST: *Calories*

4 oz. orange juice   55
1 serving of puffed wheat or puffed rice   55
with ½ cup of skim milk   45

TOTAL: 155

LUNCH:

2 oz. tuna (packed in water)   100
¼ tomato   10
⅛ head lettuce   10
with 1 oz. diet dressing   30

TOTAL: 150

DINNER:

5 oz. beef liver (broiled)   300
½ baked potato   50
6 asparagus spears   20
½ cup: beet & onion salad in vinegar   35

TOTAL: 405

TOTAL CALORIES FOR THIS DAY: 710

If desired, or for variety, you may substitute 6 oz. broiled chicken
instead of the liver.

FOURTH WEEK
FRIDAY

BREAKFAST: *Calories*

½ grapefruit   50
½ cup Cream of Wheat   50
with ½ cup of skim milk   45

                              TOTAL: 145

LUNCH:

Clam chowder:
8 oz. beef stock soup   55
½ cup cooked clams   78

                              TOTAL: 133

DINNER:

Shish kebab:
4 oz. beef   240
2 small onions   20
2 tomato wedges   20
4 mushroom caps   10
Pepper strips   5
¼ acorn squash   35
½ cup: green bean & onion salad   25
1 tangerine . . . . : . . .   40

                              TOTAL: 395

TOTAL CALORIES FOR THIS DAY: 673

If desired, or for variety, you may substitute 5 oz. chicken instead
of the beef.

FOURTH WEEK
SATURDAY

BREAKFAST: *Calories*

¾ cup strawberries	45
½ cup cottage cheese	100
TOTAL:	145

LUNCH:

Hot vegetable plate:

½ cup beets	30
½ cup summer squash	15
½ cup broccoli	20
¼ cup cottage cheese	50
with 1 oz. diet dressing	30
TOTAL:	145

DINNER:

Tuna casserole	310
Salad as follows:	
½ cucumber	15
½ tomato	20
¼ onion	10
Vinegar dressing on salad	0
½ baked apple	40
TOTAL:	395

TOTAL CALORIES FOR THIS DAY: 685

If desired, or for variety, you may substitute 5 oz. broiled beef patty instead of the tuna.

FOURTH WEEK
SUNDAY

BREAKFAST: *Calories*

4 oz. orange juice	55
1 serving of puffed wheat or puffed rice	55
with ½ cup of skim milk	45
TOTAL:	155

LUNCH:

12 oz. vegetable soup with 1 oz. beef	140
TOTAL:	140

DINNER:

5 oz. broiled beef patty	300
½ baked potato	50
Large tossed salad	20
with 1 oz. diet dressing	30
TOTAL:	400

TOTAL CALORIES FOR THIS DAY: 695

If desired, or for variety, you may substitute 6 oz. chicken instead of the beef patty.

For those of you who prefer to sleep late and skip breakfast on Sundays, the following brunch menu may be substituted for breakfast *and* lunch:

SUNDAY BRUNCH: *Calories*

½ cup fresh orange juice   55
Egg-Vegetable Omelet   245
                                    TOTAL: 300

I recognize that many people will find the discipline of a limited menu very frustrating, especially if they like to experiment in the kitchen as many of us enjoy doing.

Maintaining your daily limitations does not mean you are forbidden to step outside the boundaries of the dishes I have recommended. Remember that *the crucial yardstick is calories,* and if you ingest your 700 calories per day, using your own preferred dishes, fine; the preceding recipes and menus are ideal for the dieter, but not essential. Your own alternative dishes will be equally acceptable provided you do not exceed the maximum number of calories each day and maintain a balanced spread of calorie intake over the three daily meals. For this reason, I say: go ahead if you like to experiment and create your own menu. For those of you who might like a greater variety but don't find your inspiration in the kitchen, I am including the following recipes to broaden the possibilities at your dinner table. Variety is the spice of every meal, and maintaining a restricted diet does not preclude you from serving a tempting display at dinner time!

Main meat dishes often constitute a dietary hazard because of improper preparation and selection. I recommend roasts because of their versatility and fringe benefits, but you have to be aware of the various cuts in order to get the most for your money and keep calories to a minimum. For example: one pound of rib steak (meat only) is forty-five percent fat and more than 2,000 calories. Fat-trimmed, lean, round pot roast is less than 700 calories per pound—a big difference indeed! A little serious study of various cuts, plus a serious talk with your butcher, can help you broaden your choice of meats and at the same time, cut down on your food budget, for often the high calorie cuts are the highest priced.

Economically, roasts are great, such as a large rolled roast. In its original state, it provides one meal. Cold slices later provide meat for another meal. Small pieces lost in carving can be saved as an ingredient for a shepherd pie. From a caloric as well as a financial standpoint, roasts only add up to good sense for any family, whether on a diet or not. For the dieter, one slice can be served, while the rest of the family takes more. Everyone is happy and the dieter loses that feeling of being a gustatory burden on the household!

I would like to stress at this point that steak is *not* the most advisable dish for a dieter, both from cost and calories. A slow-simmered pot roast can be less than half the calories of steak. Chuck and flank steaks are, however, ideal for dieters, but remember: the more fat you trim off prior to cooking, the less saturated fats there will be in the final dish.

The following list of common cuts of boneless, uncooked beef will give you a good idea of the fat content and the calories involved:

	Fat Content	Calories Per Pound
Flank Steak	Very Low	650
Round Steak	11%	890
Chuck Arm	14%	1000
Rump, Roundbone Sirloin, Doublebone Sirloin, Blade Steak, Chuck Rib	25-30%	1300-1500
Club Steak	36%	1700
Porterhouse, T-Bone, Hipbone Sirloin	37-39%	1700-1800
Short Plate	41%	1800
Rib (11th and 12th)	45%	2000

There are six official grades of beef in the United States. *U.S. Prime:* tender and juicy, because it comes from young cattle, the lean areas are well marbled, meaning many streaks of fat permeate the lean part, giving good flavor to the cut. *U.S. Choice:* tasty but has less fat than prime. *U.S. Good:* still lower in fat content but with acceptable tenderness and good flavor. *U.S. Standard:* comes from older cattle and requires more care in preparation to make it truly palatable. *U.S. Commercial:* needs long, slow cooking to bring out flavor and tenderness. *U.S. Utility:*

the lowest and cheapest grade, usually lean and stringy, coming from older cows.

All these grades are equally nutritious, but the cheaper grades require a different approach in cooking to insure tenderness. Oven roasts may require top quality grades of meat, but the lower grades are perfectly acceptable for those dishes where prolonged cooking time and method bring out flavor and tenderness.

We have all seen restaurants making a big thing out of "ground sirloin," an admittedly good dish when properly prepared, but in reality, ground beef is ground beef, irrespective of the cut. For casseroles, meat loaf and similar dishes, you can save money by choosing a cheaper grade of beef and having it ground after the butcher removes all fat. The ultimate taste will differ little, if any, from "ground sirloin," especially if you add your favorite spices prior to cooking.

Chuck and flank steaks can give you low calories and low cost, and with care, you can achieve all the tenderness and flavor you may be accustomed to in higher priced cuts which also, don't forget, have higher calories because of the heavier fat content.

Most butchers carry the first three grades of beef while the lower three grades are termed "commercial." However, if you request them from your butcher, he should be able to fill your order. Stress your need for certain cuts because of your dietary limitations, and ask his advice. Remember the grade and cut affect the fat content of beef. Cuts from the hind quarters of the animal are less fatty than cuts from the front part of the carcass.

As pot roast is a recommended method of cooking meat to minimize fat and conserve flavor, you will have to plan ahead for this type of dish. After trimming as much fat off as you can and, if you desire, marinating the meat, brown and simmer the meat by itself, then refrigerate overnight in the same pot.

Next day, skim off the hardened fat and continue cooking, adding the vegetables about forty-five minutes before serving. You'll have a low-calorie, delicious roast that will rate raves at the dinner table.

In browning the meat, as with *any* dish included in a low-calorie menu, use only one tablespoon of corn oil, and after browning, drain off any fat in the pot before continuing. No matter how carefully you trim fat from the meat, there will always be some that accumulates during the browning stage. Alternatively, you may brown the meat under the broiler, allowing any fat to drain off into the drip pan.

Some people cannot resist cooking vegetables such as potatoes or carrots in the fatty drippings around a pot roast. Forget this idea; vegetables soak up fat faster than paper towels! Steam your vegetables or use a double boiler. Vegetables cooked in this way are far healthier, crisper and better tasting.

Lean meats take longer to cook than the usual fatty cuts, anywhere from twenty-five to fifty percent longer in the pot. Never hurry a pot roast by turning up the flame. High heat only toughens the meat, ruining what otherwise could be a delicious meal. Slow, steady simmering brings out the best in any cut of meat, especially if you have stainless steel waterless cookware that uses a very low heat setting. Another point to remember: the leaner the beef, the less the loss through shrinkage. A lean, boneless pot roast, properly simmered very slowly, can give you three to four three-ounce servings per pound, making it truly economical.

A good basic recipe for pot roast is as follows: Use round steak, which is only eleven percent fat and 890 calories per pound.

POT ROAST

You will need:

3½ lbs. round steak, well trimmed of fat and lean	2 medium sized onions, chopped
2-3 cups salt-free bouillon	2 tbsp. fresh parsley, chopped
1 bay leaf	garlic powder to taste
1 tsp. leaf thyme, crumbled	pepper to taste
1 pkg. substitute brown sugar	prepared mustard to taste

Place a tablespoon of corn oil in a large Dutch oven and bring to high heat. Season to taste with garlic powder and pepper and rub meat all over with prepared mustard. Lower the meat in (it should sizzle loudly!) and turn quickly to cover all sides in the hot oil. Continue until all sides are browned well. Drain off the oil, lower the heat and add the bay leaf, leaf thyme, one packet substitute brown sugar, and two cups of salt-free bouillon. Cover and simmer at low heat for three hours. The liquid should not bubble rapidly, but barely boil, allowing the meat to cook gently. Check it every hour and if any liquid has boiled away, you may add up to another cup of salt-free bouillon.

Remove from heat, remove the bay leaf and refrigerate overnight. An hour before you plan to serve the roast, scrape off the solidified fat from the top of the liquid and discard. Add two chopped onions and two tablespoons chopped parsley. Place on a low flame and simmer for about forty-five minutes.

Each three-ounce serving of this pot roast contains less than 200 calories, making it an ideal for substitution in the diet plan outlined instead of the specified meat dishes.

An interesting variation on an old French recipe shows how a hefty dash of imagination can come up with a dish that is (I have since discovered) a very popular recipe in the Cape section of South Africa, where it is called Dutch Burgundy Beef.

DUTCH BURGUNDY BEEF

You will need:

3½ lbs. lean, well trimmed of fat, round steak	1 cup onion, chopped
1 tsp. poultry seasoning	1 cup carrots, sliced
1 tsp. pumpkin pie spice	1 cup fresh mushrooms, sliced
½ tsp. grated orange rind	½ cup Burgundy wine
½ tsp. grated lemon rind	2½ cups salt-free bouillon
2 tsps. fresh parsley, chopped	

Prepare the meat as in the preceding pot roast recipe. After browning and pouring off the cooking oil, add the following:

poultry seasoning, pumpkin pie spice, grated orange rind, grated lemon rind, fresh parsley, chopped onion, sliced carrots, sliced fresh mushrooms, Burgundy wine, salt-free beef bouillon. Simmer very gently for three hours. Remove and refrigerate overnight. An hour before serving skim off the fat from the top of the liquid, place back on heat and simmer for a half hour.

A three-ounce serving contains less than 240 calories.

NEW ENGLAND POT ROAST

You will need:

3½ lbs. chuck arm roast, boneless and trimmed of fat

3 cups salt-free beef bouillon

2 bay leaves

1 tsp. poultry seasoning

3 large stalks of celery, scraped and cut into six inch lengths

4 large carrots, peeled and sliced

2 medium turnips, peeled and sliced

2 tsps. salt-free soy sauce

The traditional New England pot roast is bland, but the following recipe can be made truly tasty by adding two teaspoons of salt-free soy sauce.

Prepare the meat as in the preceding recipes. After pouring off the oil add the salt-free beef bouillon, bay leaves, and poultry seasoning. Simmer gently for three hours. Refrigerate and a half hour before serving, remove the solidified fat from the top of the liquid, and add the celery, carrots, and turnips. Simmer for twenty minutes.

One three-ounce serving contains less than 200 calories.

SHANGHAI POT ROAST

You will need:

3½ lbs. boneless, chuck arm, trimmed of all fat
1 tbsp. corn oil
1 cup dry sherry
1 cup salt-free beef bouillon
5 tbsp. salt-free soy sauce
1 tbsp. ground ginger
½ tsp. pepper
1 tsp. dry mustard
½ tsp. sweet basil

1 cup water
1 medium sized onion
1 cup bean sprouts
½ cup water chestnuts
1 cup peapods

Marinade:
2 cloves fresh garlic, mashed
salt-free soy sauce to cover
pepper to taste

Cover meat with marinade and allow to stand for a half hour. Remove meat from marinade and brown in one tablespoon of hot corn oil. Drain and add the dry sherry, salt-free beef bouillon, salt-free soy sauce, ground ginger, pepper, dry mustard, and sweet basil. Simmer gently for three hours, then refrigerate overnight.

An hour before serving, skim the solidified fat from the top of the liquid and place back on a low flame. Blend in a blender one cup of water and one onion (you may chop the onion by hand if you prefer) and add to the pot, together with the bean sprouts, water chestnuts and peapods. Cook gently for twenty minutes, then serve. The meat and vegetable mixture is especially good over rice. A three-ounce portion of meat with a tablespoon of vegetables and gravy contains less than 200 calories.

For those who like Italian food, the following is especially good.

LOW-CAL STEAK ROMANO

You will need:

1½ lb. flank steak, sliced ½ inch thick	1 tbsp. corn oil
1 tbsp. grated Romano cheese	1 lb. fresh tomatoes
	1 cup water
1¼ tsp. oregano	1 medium onion
½ tsp. garlic powder	fine string or twine

Make several crosscuts on the pieces of meat, about halfway through, and spread with the following: one tablespoon grated Romano cheese, one teaspoon oregano, one half teaspoon garlic powder, and one-quarter teaspoon pepper. Roll each piece of meat into a sausage shape and tie firmly every couple of inches with fine string or white twine. Nylon thread is also good, wrapped around like a mesh to enclose the meat and hold it in shape.

Place corn oil in a deep pan or Dutch oven and heat till fairly hot. Drop the meat in and roll it around until well browned on all sides. Drain off the oil.

Liquefy in a blender one pound of fresh peeled tomatoes, one onion, and one cup of water. Add one-quarter teaspoon oregano, and one half teaspoon pepper. Pour over meat, cover and simmer gently for two hours.

Remove the meat and place on a serving platter. Continue simmering the sauce until thick.

Remove the strings from the meat and pour the sauce over the meat. This amount should provide six three ounce servings. Total calories per three-ounce portion: under 200.

For generations people have looked upon shepherd pie as a convenient means of using up leftover meats, and as such, a way to stretch the family food budget. However, shepherd pie deserves a better status than being a catch-all for scraps from your roast! This dish, properly prepared, can be a tingling taste treat for everyone in the family, and one which is well within the dieter's limitations. In addition to being a worthy main dish for dinner, shepherd pie can be used the next day in a variety of ways including thin slices for sandwiches and warmed with gravy for a hot luncheon dish.

SHEPHERD PIE

You will need:

leftover roast meat scraps	mashed potatoes to cover
2 egg whites	chopped parsley
1 medium sized onion, finely chopped	pepper to taste
	salt-free soy sauce to taste

You will also need to have your own meat grinder to prepare the meat. You can use the higher-priced electric models, or do very well with a hand grinder that sells for less than ten dollars. The savings in meal preparation make a meat grinder a worthy investment.

Take all your leftover pieces from a roast and grind them up; then add the egg whites, pepper and a dash of salt-free soy sauce. Stir until thoroughly mixed into a smooth paste; then spread over the bottom of a casserole dish. The thickness of the meat should be not less than two inches over the bottom of the dish. Spread the chopped onion over the surface of the meat. Then cover with well-mashed baked or boiled potatoes, about an inch thick. An interesting design can be made by drawing a fork gently over the top of the mashed potatoes.

Place in a hot oven (350-375 degrees) for thirty minutes, or until the top of the mashed potatoes is lightly browned. Be sure and stand the casserole in a pan of water about an inch deep during cooking to prevent the bottom (meat) part of the pie from drying out. Before serving, sprinkle chopped parsley over the top.

A three-ounce serving contains less than 200 calories.

Frequently dieters look upon stews as automatically fattening, which they need not be if properly prepared. The following recipe gives you a delicious main dish with only 220 calories per three-ounce serving, and has the advantage of being frozen in small aluminum pans for individual servings at any time.

2 lbs. very lean boneless round steak, well trimmed of fat
1 tbsp. salt-free soy sauce
1 cup wheat germ
1 tbsp. corn oil
1 cup sherry
2 cups salt-free beef bouillon
1 cup carrots, diced
2 large onions, sliced
1 cup fresh mushrooms, sliced
½ cup celery, chopped
½ cup green peas
½ tsp. salt
¼ tsp. pepper
large brown paper bag

Cut the meat into small cubes about an inch square and toss in a bowl with a tablespoon of salt-free soy sauce so that each piece of meat is thinly coated with the sauce.

Place the wheat germ in a large brown paper sack, add the meat, and shake well to coat each cube with wheat germ. You should hold one hand beneath the sack during shaking to prevent possible tearing.

Have a large Dutch oven ready on the stove with a tablespoon of corn oil, heated fairly hot. Drop in the meat and stir quickly with a wooden spoon until each piece is nicely seared. Add the following: sherry, salt-free beef bouillon, diced carrots, sliced onions, sliced mushrooms, chopped celery, green peas, salt, pepper, and garlic salt. Bring to a boil, then turn down the heat and simmer gently for two hours.

Refrigerate overnight, and next day, simmer again for another hour before serving, by which time the stew should be thick and rich.

For a spicy East Indian difference, you may turn the above stew into a beef curry by merely adding two teaspoons of curry powder thirty minutes before serving. For those unaccustomed to curries, I suggest you go carefully with the curry powder until you determine the degree of spiciness you prefer. Some people like a very "hot" curry, others enjoy it on the bland side.

Either way, plain or curried, this stew is delicious and contains less than 200 calories per three-ounce serving.

A low-calorie, economical version of beef strogonoff can be added to your menu with the following recipe, which is a guaranteed taste-teaser.

BEEF BALLS STROGONOFF

You will need:

2 lbs. very lean ground beef	1 tsp. salt-free soy sauce
2 egg whites	1 tsp. parsley, chopped
½ cup onion, finely chopped	1 cup mushrooms,
½ cup wheat germ	finely chopped
2 tsp. prepared mustard	¼ tsp. sweet basil
2 cups salt-free beef bouillon	¼ cup sherry
¼ tsp. pepper	1 cup cottage cheese, blended

Combine meat in a bowl with two egg whites. (I should stress that in binding meat for cooking, the white of an egg is all that is necessary. The yolk only adds calories and cholesterol, both unnecessary for the dieter). Add the following: chopped fresh onion, wheat germ, one teaspoon prepared mustard. Mix together thoroughly and take about a dessert spoon of the mixture and roll it into a small meat ball between your hands. Continue to roll all the meat into small balls, placing them in a wide casserole which has been sprayed with lecithin to prevent sticking. Place in a hot oven (400 degrees) until the meat balls are slightly browned, but not cooked all the way through.

Add together: salt-free beef bouillon, pepper, salt-free soy sauce, one teaspoon mustard, chopped parsley or parsley flakes, finely chopped mushrooms, and sweet basil. This mixture should be well stirred and poured over the browned meat balls.

Allow to simmer gently in the oven for about an hour at 350 degrees. Before serving, remove the meat balls into a separate dish, and add to the sauce the following: sherry, and blended cottage cheese. Stir well, replace the meat balls and put back in the oven for fifteen minutes with the heat turned *off*. This recipe makes eight to ten servings of approximately 170 calories each.

We've been talking mostly about beef, the traditional meat for most Americans, but there are other tasty dishes that do not involve beef. For example, veal—which is one of the lowest calorie meats you can buy, and as such, is ideal for the dieter's menu. Although many people object to the blandness of veal compared with beef, you can perk up any veal dish by the addition of spices. In fact, you can easily avoid the "sameness" usually associated with a strict diet by experimenting with spices and with various ways of preparing your menus. My only stipulation is in always counting your calories. Imagination and a shelf of spices can work wonders for a tired appetite!

Why not try veal with a Chinese flavor!

CHINESE SWEET-AND-SOUR VEAL

You will need:

1½ lbs. veal shoulder	1 cup celery, chopped
1 tbsp. corn oil	½ cup bean sprouts
1 cup salt-free beef bouillon	1 tbsp. wine vinegar
½ cup onion, finely chopped	3 tbsp. salt-free soy sauce
1 medium sized can	2 tsp. arrowroot
unsweetened pineapple	pepper to taste
chunks with juice	

Cut the meat into small cubes and brown in a skillet using one tablespoon corn oil. Add: salt-free beef bouillon, finely chopped onion, unsweetened pineapple chunks, including the juice and simmer for forty-five minutes.

Now add: chopped celery, bean sprouts, wine vinegar, salt-free soy sauce, arrowroot, and a dash of pepper to taste. Simmer gently for ten minutes and serve. This recipe makes about six servings of 275 calories each.

Wine lends itself very well to veal dishes, adding that gourmet touch without adding calories. The following dish tastes like a million dollars—rich and delicious—but with only 260 calories per three-ounce serving.

VEAL STEW

You will need:

2 lb. veal shoulder	½ cup celery, chopped
1 tbsp. corn oil	1 cup sherry
½ cup onion, chopped	½ tsp. fresh lemon juice
1 clove garlic, minced	¼ tsp. pepper
1 lb. fresh mushrooms, sliced	1 bay leaf
	chopped parsley

Cut the veal into one-inch cubes and brown in one tablespoon of corn oil. Add: chopped onion, garlic, mushrooms, and celery. Stir gently while cooking for about three minutes. Now add the sherry, lemon juice, pepper, and bay leaf. Simmer gently for one hour. Remove the bay leaf and serve hot with a sprinkling of chopped parsley over the top.

And here's another savory 260 calorie-per-serving dish with veal.

VEAL ROLLS MILANESE

You will need:

1½ lb. veal	½ tsp. poultry seasoning
4 oz. chopped beef (fresh, not cooked)	3 tbsp. fresh tomato, peeled and liquefied
4 hardboiled egg whites, mashed	1 tsp. corn oil
½ cup onion, minced	1 tsp. fresh lemon juice
4 tbsp. parsley, chopped	twine

Slice the veal thin into six to eight pieces.
Combine the beef, mashed hard-boiled egg whites, onion,

chopped parsley, poultry seasoning, and liquefied fresh tomatoes.

Spread the mixture evenly over the strips of veal, then roll up and tie with twine or nylon thread. Place them seam-side-down in a shallow baking dish and brush the tops with a mixture of half corn oil, half lemon juice. Cover and bake in a moderate oven (350 degrees) for one hour.

In your experimenting with new recipes of your own, don't overlook veal as a replacement for beef in a meat loaf. And scraps from a veal roast also help cut calories in a shepherd pie that is particularly good cold.

For another change of pace without adding excessive calories to your menu, try lamb. Many people reject lamb because they claim it is too fatty, a false notion stemming from lamb chops which are, admittedly, high in calories no matter how you cook them. BUT . . . unlike beef, where fat is distributed throughout the tissue, lamb fat is mainly on the outside, enabling your butcher (or yourself) to trim away the fat, leaving only the lean meat. A leg of lamb, properly trimmed, is one of the leanest meats you can buy, and, in our opinion, a welcome taste change from beef.

Don't pass over lamb as something you should avoid. For any diet, properly prepared lamb contributes minimal calories compared with other meats, plus a distinctive flavor that has made lamb a traditional dish in England and the Middle East.

LAMB SHISH KEBAB

You will need:

1 lb. lean lamb leg	*Marinade:*
tomato wedges	½ cup water
quartered onions	2 tsp. salt-free soy sauce
sliced green peppers	¼ tsp. thyme
corn oil	½ tsp. grated lemon rind
	3 tbsp. fresh lemon juice
	¼ tsp. crushed rosemary
	1 clove garlic, pressed

Cut the lamb into one-inch squares. Place in a deep bowl and marinate for two to four hours.

Spear the meat on to a skewer, alternating the lamb with tomato wedges, small quartered onions, and slices of green pepper. Broil for twenty minutes, turning every five minutes, and brushing the meat with a little corn oil. The meat and vegetables should be nicely browned when ready. Slide off the skewer on to a plate and serve with a tossed salad.

Delicious, and only 200 calories a three-ounce serving.

Because of its flavor, lamb is particularly well suited to curries. For a change of pace, try the following, which contains only 280 calories per serving.

LAMB NEW DELHI

You will need:

1 lb. roast leg of lamb	1/2 tsp. ground ginger
3 tbsp. onion, chopped	1 tsp. salt-free soy sauce
1/2 tsp. garlic powder	2 cups fresh tomatoes,
1 tsp. curry powder	peeled and liquefied

Place the roast lamb leg cut into one-inch cubes in a large saucepan together with the chopped onion, garlic powder, curry powder, ground ginger, salt-free soy sauce, and liquefied fresh tomatoes.

Simmer for twenty minutes, gently. Serve very hot.

Like all stew-type dishes, curry improves with overnight refrigeration and warming up the next day.

A Turkish version of exotic meat balls is made with lamb, and tastes very rich, yet has only 220 calories per three ounce serving.

MEAT BALLS YEMEN

You will need:

2 lb. trimmed ground lamb	¾ tbsp. garlic powder
4 egg whites	2 tsp. brewers yeast
2 fresh medium sized tomatoes, peeled and liquefied	½ cup wheat germ
	1 tsp. cinnamon
	3 cups low-cal yogurt
1 cup parsley, chopped	paprika to taste

Combine in a bowl: freshly ground lamb, egg whites, tomatoes, chopped parsley, garlic powder, brewers yeast, wheat germ, and cinnamon. Blend together thoroughly and roll into small meat balls, about one to two inches in diameter. Place the meat balls under the broiler until browned on all sides, then arrange in a deep casserole and cover with low-cal yogurt that has been gently warmed in a double broiler. (Do not allow the yogurt to boil!) Sprinkle with paprika and chopped parsley and serve at once.

In buying lamb, remember the following tips: a leg of lamb is excellent, provided your butcher trims off *all* the fat. Alternatively, you can have the butcher trim the fat, remove the bone and make up a rolled lamb roast. For barbecue or pan frying, use only the lean lamb chops cut from the leg. For stews, use the lean portion from the leg, although a shoulder roast, well trimmed, is a little cheaper and works just as well. For ground lamb, as with ground beef, the cut makes no difference as long as all fat is trimmed off before cooking.

Taste tip: lamb in any form goes very well with sliced baked apples, artificially sweetened apple sauce, or cranberry sauce.

Now let's talk about chicken, which is possibly one of the most economical and versatile meats obtainable. A word of warning, however: for chicken dishes that involve cooking in a pot on top of the stove rather than baking in the oven, be sure to strip off the skin, which is where most of the fat is found.

A tablespoon of chicken fat adds around 125 calories—unnecessary in *any* diet! This inherent fat that surrounds the chicken is what enables you to roast a chicken without adding any oil or butter. However, do not attempt to roast a chicken that has been skinned, otherwise you'll wind up with an unappealing hard crust over the bird! Skinned chicken can be broiled, and also works very well in stews and casseroles.

One of my most popular recipes for chicken is the following which makes six servings at only 220 calories each, and with a flavor straight out of a Polynesian luau!

CHICKEN HAWAIIAN

You will need:

3 lbs. skinned chicken breasts	4 tbsp. green pepper, finely chopped
1 cup mushrooms, sliced	3 tbsp. dry sherry
1 medium sized onion, finely chopped	½ cup water
1 cup orange juice	½ tsp. pepper
1 tsp. orange peel, finely grated	2 tsp. parsley, chopped
	1 tbsp. arrowroot

Place chicken in a shallow baking dish. Cover with one cup of sliced mushrooms and a sauce made from the following ingredients, simmered over low heat until thick: onion, finely chopped, orange juice, finely grated orange peel, finely chopped green peppers, dry sherry, water, pepper chopped parsley, and arrowroot for thickening.

After covering the chicken with the sauce, bake in a moderate oven (350 degrees) for an hour to an hour and a half, basting frequently. In place of basting, you may cover the baking dish completely with aluminum foil, sealing the edges, for the first forty-five minutes of cooking. Basting, however, results in better flavor through the chicken and a tastier dish.

For a variation, you may substitute crushed unsweetened pineapple for the orange in the recipe.

Chicken a la King seems to have gained the questionable reputation as being merely a means of serving up leftover chicken; but with a little imagination, you can make a variety of tempting dishes from the basic recipe, which is good for eight to ten servings of only 240 calories each.

CHICKEN A LA KING

You will need:

4 cups cooked, skinless chicken, chopped	¼ tsp. sweet basil
1 cup salt-free chicken bouillon	½ cup skim milk
	4 hard boiled egg whites
¼ tsp. pepper	¼ cup arrowroot
¼ tsp. thyme	1 tbsp. corn oil margarine
	1 cup onion, finely chopped

Place one tablespoon of corn oil margarine in a skillet and add finely chopped fresh onion. Cook over gentle heat for fifteen minutes. The margarine should not be hot enough to brown the onion, but merely to cook it without scorching or until transparent. The onions should be cooked, but still clear and clean looking. Now add the following: chopped, cooked, skinless chicken breasts, salt-free chicken bouillon, pepper, thyme, sweet basil, and simmer gently for one minute. Mix together in a blender the following: skim milk, hardboiled egg whites and arrowroot. Pour together and cook gently until the mixture bubbles and thickens, about two minutes. Serve over rice.

At your discretion, you may add: chopped parsely; chopped celery; a cup of sliced mushrooms; chopped green peppers; sliced pimientos; or two tablespoons dry sherry for a gourmet flavor. Let your imagination run riot and turn your Chicken a la King into a dish that really tickles the palate, and remember what we said about spices: they add only flavor, but no calories.

Finally, there is fish, something we cannot stress too highly in a dieter's menu. Nothing is lower in fat and higher in protein than whitefish, when properly prepared. Restaurants are notorious for soaking fish in batter, heavy in starch and absorbed cooking fat, or drowing fish in a rich sauce overloaded with calories.

But at less than 400 calories per pound, whitefish has no competition as a valuable food source that's ideal for the dieter. The following recipes have proved outstanding favorites among my patients, and are not only low in calories but economical as well.

HALIBUT

You will need:

1 lb. fresh halibut fillets	10 mushrooms, chopped
¼ tsp. pepper	1 tomato, sliced
¼ tsp. paprika	chopped parsley for garnish
1 lemon, peeled and chopped	

Cut fresh halibut fillets in convenient sized pieces. Place in a shallow baking dish. Shake over the fish: pepper, and paprika. Cover with a mixture of chopped, peeled lemon and chopped mushrooms. Place a slice of tomato on each piece of fish and sprinkle with chopped parsley. Cover completely with aluminum foil and bake at 400 degrees for ten minutes; remove the foil and continue baking for another twenty minutes. Serve hot from the oven. This makes four servings at only 160 calories each.

ITALIAN STYLE WHITEFISH

You will need:

1½ lbs. fresh whitefish (flounder or perch)	3-4 cups cooked spinach, chopped and well drained
1 tbsp. arrowroot	¼ cup Parmesan cheese, grated
2 lemons	pepper to taste

Cut the fish into small pieces and arrange in small clumps in a deep baking dish. I suggest you spray the dish with lecithin to prevent sticking.

Sprinkle with pepper and douse with lemon juice. Cover with aluminum foil and bake in a moderate oven (350 degrees) for fifteen minutes, by which time the fish should just flake easily when tested with a fork. Pour off the liquid (the water, lemon juice, and fish nutrients) into a small saucepan. If necessary, add water to make about three-fourths cup of liquid. Bring to a boil and stir in enough arrowroot (about one tablespoon) to thicken it. Remove from heat.

Now take cooked chopped spinach and arrange around the clumps of fish in the baking dish, pour over the sauce and top with grated Parmesan cheese. Pop into a hot oven (425 degrees) for about five minutes, or until the sauce is bubbling. Remove and serve at once.

If desired, another green vegetable such as broccoli or green beans may be substituted for the spinach.

This recipe tastes terribly rich and yields six servings which have the delightful bonus of only 135 calories each.

STUFFED FLOUNDER

You will need:

2 lbs. fresh flounder fillets (8 pieces)	3/4 cup cottage cheese, blended
3/4 cup mushrooms, chopped	3/4 cup water
3 tbsp. onion, minced	1/4 cup dry white wine
1 7 1/2 oz. can of crabmeat, drained and chopped	3 tbsp. arrowroot
1 tbsp. parsley chopped	1/2 cup shredded dry cottage cheese
1/4 tsp. pepper	paprika to taste

Spread flounder fillets out flat and trimmed into 8 pieces. Over each fillet spread the following which should be thoroughly mixed in a bowl before spreading on the fish: chopped mushrooms, minced onion, crabmeat, drained and chopped, chopped parsley, and pepper. After spreading evenly, roll each flounder piece and place seam-side-down on a baking dish. Any excess stuffing mixture can be placed around each fillet.

Now prepare a sauce as follows in a small sauce pan: blended cottage cheese, water, dry white wine, and arrowroot for thickening. Stir while the sauce thickens over a low flame, then add shredded dry cottage cheese. Continue stirring until the cheese melts. Pour over the flounder fillets, top lightly with paprika and bake in a hot oven (400 degrees) for thirty minutes, or until the flounder flakes easily when tested with a fork.

This recipe serves eight people at only slightly more than 180 calories per servings.

Whitefish need not be poached or steamed to keep down the calories. You can oven-fry any whitefish by rolling it in a little wheat germ, with a little pepper, and baking in the oven at 450 degrees for about twelve minutes, or until the fish flakes when tested with a fork. A serving of sole, flounder, or perch cooked in this manner adds up to only 140 calories.

The preceding section dealing with meat, poultry, and fish should indicate how you have the freedom to dream up any type of dish your gourmet taste desires, provided you stick within the caloric limitations of your diet. I have purposely not included vegetable or salad dishes, as I feel this is an individual matter. Some people prefer just a salad; others enjoy a vegetable, cooked, with the meal instead. However, I'll pass this tip along as an aid in keeping your daily menu varied and interesting: instead of serving *one* vegetable (such as string beans), place a small portion of three or more vegetables in the pot, making an appealing looking and varied tasting combination.

You doubtless have seen these combinations in the frozen food locker at the supermarket such as "Vegetables Italiano" or "Vegetables Hawaiian," and usually at somewhat higher prices than the individual items sold separately. Why not make up your own combinations? The governing factor should be visual and the taste interesting: for example, try to include one yellow vegetable (carrots or squash) and one "leaf" type green vegetable (broccoli). This gives you a dish that is interesting to look at, and delicious to eat, and most certainly a change from the usual plain dish of a single vegetable. There are numerous combinations that can be used: cauliflower, peas, and crookneck squash, or broccoli, carrots, Italian green beans, and mushrooms. Go to it and let your imagination run wild. You'll find mealtimes become more interesting and appetizing, helping to remove the psychological resistance to a "diet."

Simple meals can become boring for the dieter, introducing a stress factor which can sometimes prejudice a person against staying on the prescribed diet for any length of time, BUT . . .

if the appearance and variety of dishes is stimulating, there is a constant enjoyment and interest in mealtimes, even though the portions may be less than one might otherwise consume.

There is no reason why you should not enjoy your meals while cutting down on your calories, and using the recipes in this chapter, plus any you can dream up yourself, will maintain your enthusiasm and interest.

You will note that salt has been excluded from these recipes. This is because salt holds water and retards an even weight loss. I recommend using salt substitute, *but only after cooking;* if you try to cook with salt substitute, you'll wind up with a very bitter tasting dish!

Of course, no matter how much you may enjoy your food, the greatest enjoyment in store will come from seeing those unwanted extra pounds melt away week after week, and staying off *permanently,* which they certainly will do if you follow my guidelines completely and do not exceed your daily caloric limitations.

Remember the Sixth Commandment of Psychostructure: *My daily diet must not exceed 700 calories, and every day I must record everything I eat as well as weigh myself.*

7. MILK, BREAD, AND ALCOHOL

MILK

I want to take this opportunity to voice my feelings on what I consider one of the most scurrilous advertising campaigns in the country today: namely, the gigantic (and unfortunately successful) promotion by the American Dairy Council to coerce every man, woman, and child to deluge their stomachs with milk morning, noon, and night.

As I have mentioned before, milk is outstanding as a food for baby cows; as for being nature's most perfect food, I say: bull!

Milk is far from being the perfect food for humans. It lacks iron. It contains large amounts of cholesterol. It contains large amounts of sodium, so if you happen to be a heart patient with bad teeth, it may do you some good, but at the expense of your heart. And for those of us concerned about overweight, milk contains a high number of calories. Do you wonder now why I am adamantly opposed to milk being included in the average diet?

Man is the only animal that drinks milk after being weaned. This is a habit stemming from tradition, and aggravated by the daily urging of the Dairy Council's massive advertising campaign. Believe me, milk is *not* good for every body—particularly over-weight bodies!

Animals, including cows, do not drink milk after being weaned and get along just fine. Humans can do the same, for there is nothing in milk that we cannot get from other items in our diet.

Maybe a little information on calcium metabolism will ex-plain why I take this view about milk in the diet. First, the body contains calcium in the largest amounts in the teeth and the bones. There is some in the muscles, and some in the blood which helps with the clotting mechanism. If all the teeth and bones in a person's body were ground up, you would have a small pile of calcium; this total calcium content of the body structure equals the amount of calcium in a very few quarts of milk.

Most of the calcium ingested in milk finds its way into the urine and is excreted. You retain hardly any calcium from drink-ing milk as an adult, and all the adult calcium needs are con-tained in other foods. There is no need to think you'll wind up with a calcium deficiency if you stop drinking milk. The only thing that will happen, if you suffer from obesity, is that you will be cutting down on your calories when you stop drinking milk, and thereby taking a very positive step towards gaining control of your weight.

Contrary to the general belief, three glases of milk a day is far in excess of the needed calcium for the body. If you are a parent or grandparent, remember this: milk is for baby cows, *not* for weaned, growing humans, especially if they happen to have a weight problem.

Many mothers ladle out a glass of milk to their children when the young'uns are thirsty, thereby setting in motion a truly disastrous chain of events. For the child who has a tendency towards fat, the Constance Bannister chubby baby type especially, milk is unfortunately the one item that sees the most action at the kitchen table. No matter if junior refuses to eat his food, or turns away from cookies and pie, as long as he gulps down that glass of milk, his mother feels satisfied that he won't develop signs of malnutrition. She fails to realize that she is only planting the seeds of obesity in later years, a condition that can well compound other health problems. Remember: milk should be regarded as a *food, not* as something to quench thirst.

Let's bury another myth: iced tea or coffee, especially de-caffeinated coffee, is *not* bad for kids. It does not stunt their growth or rot their teeth. Far better for junior to quench his thirst with iced tea or coffee or lemonade with artificial sweetners than to get into the habit of drinking milk, which is just as bad for him as Coca-cola or other high calorie liquids.

For those of you who feel they cannot drink their coffee black (which I strongly recommend), you may add skim milk which contains the lowest calories of the milk products.

But in general, for those of you who are fighting a lifelong battle of the bulge, and for our children who have a similar problem, milk should be outlawed from the table. If you're counting your calories, count milk out of your diet. As for milk products, cottage cheese is the *only* one acceptable. The rest—OUT!!

BREAD

Bread is traditionally the staff of life. We talk about earning our daily bread. The counter-culture today refers to "bread" as essential for existence, and while those using this term refer to money, the underlying inference is the same: that bread is essential to our survival. Bread is so ingrained in our consciousness that the following statement is, I know, going to be hard to take, but it happens to be true: bread is the Number One cause of problems for people who tend to be obese. Number One? you say incredulously, what possible harm could a single slice of bread be to one's diet?

I'll tell you. Because you never have a single slice of bread. Bread is a lonely thing. A slice never is seen in public by itself; it always has another with it. Two slices. And bread is so modest that it's always dressed, usually *over*-dressed in a variety of calorie-laden spreads like mayonnaise, peanut butter, and grape jelly.

Bread is always on the table, and most of us eat it because

it's there, and for no other reason. As far as I'm concerned, bread is only something to keep the grease off your fingers when you eat a piece of pastrami!

The average American eats between four and six slices of bread a day. Let's assume an average of 100 calories per slice—that means an average of 500 calories per day. Do you know what that means? It means, pure and simple: FIFTY pounds a year. If you had not eaten bread for the past year, and were the average individual, you would be FIFTY pounds lighter today.

As a positive reinforcement, along with keeping your diary and daily weight, conduct a funeral for bread. Take a loaf into the yard and bury it with all the ceremony you can dream up. On top of the grave, place a marker—"BREAD IS DEAD"—and firmly resolve you will never again eat a slice of bread.

At first you will go through all the painful stages of losing a best friend. You will feel denial at first, then hostility, and finally resignation. You will doubtless direct a number of very uncomplimentary comments at me, but let's face it: you *must* understand that if you are going to solve your weight problem permanently, and achieve that slender body you yearn for, there are certain things you *have* to *do,* and certain things you *have to do without.*

Bread, and any of its varied and tempting forms, is to be relegated to the past. One day when you remember how terribly overweight you used to be, you may also recall the mouth-watering taste of your favorite sandwich, but so what? Isn't the trim figure in the mirror more than enough compensation?

ALCOHOL

Just as excessive advertising by the Dairy Council has helped turn us into a nation of milk guzzlers, so also is the liquor industry to blame for the false glamor attached to drinks containing alcohol, prompting too many people to regard a cocktail as the key to joining the ranks of the beautiful people. For those of us with an obesity problem, alcohol can help turn us into anything *but* a beautiful person! I've heard it said too many times that there are no fat alcoholics. I disagree. I happen to know quite a number of alcoholics who are grossly overweight, among them many who have proudly proclaimed they have gone on "the drinking man's diet." Let me say right now: for anyone on any type of diet to lose weight, alcohol is *out. No alcohol.* Why? It's very simple: alcohol is a highly concentrated type of food with a very high caloric content. Compare six ounces of steak (360 calories) with six ounces of alcohol (100 proof vodka—500 calories). If you are going to compare the satisfaction you get from either, that is another matter; so perhaps a few facts about alcohol will be in order for the dieter to understand the very real dangers of ingesting alcohol.

Let's strip those glamorous sounding drinks of their names and take a look at the major ingredient of every potion served at a bar: namely, alcohol. Technically, *ethyl alcohol,* which consists of six carbon atoms, six hydrogen atoms, and one oxygen atom, combined into a substance that has very unique properties when ingested into the human body.

In brief, alcohol is a stimulant *and* a depressant for the central nervous system. After you imbibe a certain quantity of alcohol, it is absorbed by the fat cells in the brain, thereby altering the mental processes. Reaction time is slowed, judgment is impaired, and a host of emotional changes occur after alcohol is absorbed. Unfortunately man decided centuries ago that an alcoholic drink eases the daily pressures of living, but as we all know, either from personal experience or observation, this is not the best way to ease pressures. In fact, for someone suffering from obesity, it is a highly dangerous practice.

Why?

Because to maintain your regimen and your diet, you need a constantly conscious effort not to fall *off* your diet and go on an eating binge, which is why drinking binges and eating binges usually go hand-in-hand. Even when you're sober, or minus any tranquilizer or drug, you occasionally will experience an episode of unstructured eating. This is to be expected; it's part of the routine because none of us is perfect, and there *will* be those moments when we slip. That's when we're sober, remember; but when you're drinking, the danger lies not only in the calories consumed, but more significantly, in the loss of your conscious intellectual guard against overeating. This is the major problem with alcohol for the dieter: becoming careless and losing your awareness of what you may and may not eat.

So if you have taken a drink to ease the pressure after a bad day at the office, you find, inevitably, that the pressure is still there. You have gained nothing except those extra pounds from the calories in the drinks, plus however much forbidden food you have consumed while in a euphoric alcoholic haze. So, I say again: for the dieter, alcohol is *out*.

There is another myth I want to dispel: that the calories in alcohol are somehow unique, and are burned up and are not converted to fat. Not true. Do not be deluded into thinking that alcohol does not convert itself into fat. It does. A calorie is a calorie, whether it comes in a martini or a mushroom omelette, and any calories not consumed by an outlay of energy by the body will be converted to fat.

Another fact I have gleaned from my years of obesity research: most people with a weight problem seldom drink alcohol as the purist does. From a recent survey on obese people who drink, it was revealed that their favorite libation was a Brandy Alexander with ice cream! That's about 700 calories in *one drink* —the same number you are allowed for an entire day on your diet. Does anyone dare to say now that one drink can't do you any harm?

There are other very serious health problems related to alcohol and dieting: for example, if you are in a fasting or a semi-starvation state, your liver becomes very susceptible to damage, and if you go on a diet that is deficient in vitamins and amino acids, you run a grave risk of damaging your liver.

Many times people develop an allergic response to alcohol without knowing it, and when they go on a diet where the vitamins and amino acids that protect the liver are deficient, they can do irreparable harm to the liver through daily drinking.

There are several stages to the development of cirrhosis of the liver. Almost all obese men and women have a fatty infiltration of the liver. Following the stage of cell breakdown called *sitolisis,* comes *fibrosis* which comes from overindulgence in alcohol, and no amount of abstinence, vitamins, or treatment will reverse the process, and you're left with permanent liver damage. In the terminal stages of cirrhosis, most people are no longer fat; they become scrawny, scraggly-necked, bleary-eyed—the stereotype of the Bowery bum, but this is hardly an ideal way to lose weight!

I've said: NO ALCOHOL. But, and I am being practical now, there are times when you want to take a drink. If you decide you simply *must* have a drink, for whatever reason, at least choose the one alcoholic beverage that has the least calories: wine. Chianti, with its low sugar content, and cabernet sauvignon or pinot chardonnay are low in calories. Order by the glass, and never by the bottle. As I say, if you *must* have a drink, perhaps for a special occasion once a year, this would be permissible. But on a daily basis, you can do enduring damage to yourself by taking that drink. Even one cocktail before dinner every evening will mean *ten* pounds a year you automatically add on to your weight. It's the little things that count when restricting your diet, and drinking is one of them.

Let me give you another example of my practical nature in regard to alcohol: I am quite aware that many businessmen and women are obliged to attend cocktail parties as part of their job. It has been said that more deals are closed over the glass in the hand than the glass on a desk. How do you endure an endless round of cocktail parties and luncheon gatherings without being weeded out as a wet blanket for refusing to take a drink? Many a pall is cast over the proceedings by someone proclaiming their abstinence from alcohol. What can you do?

The answer is very simple. You carry round a glass of diet soda and no one will know the difference! And if it's a business meeting with a client, don't feel you're *persona non grata* at the local bar if you don't order liquor. Tavern owners make more money from abstainers than drinkers because you're still charged a high price for your glass of soda, and the bartender still gets a good tip from you. Don't be shy about ordering just what you should: namely, something that *looks* like a drink, but which contains no alcohol. You'll be ahead of the game, both in keeping down your calories and keeping up your mental alertness by not having a brain clouded by a cocktail!

As for social parties where there is a bar set up and an hors d'oeuvre table: position yourself as far as possible away from food and drink, and remember Stuelke's Law of the Cocktail Party: "The distance from the hors d'oeuvre table is inversely proportional to your weight." Stay as far as possible from food and drinks, and embroil yourself in constant conversation. If you're in a position to reach out for a snack, you're going to! Remove yourself from temptation and you'll be more likely to stay out of trouble.

Remember that your status with your friends or business associates need not depend upon your consumption of food or drink. In fact, you'll find your status rising considerably after you've lost weight and are able to maintain a slender, healthy figure—a constant tribute to your perseverance, dedication, and ability to set yourself a goal and achieve it: certainly three qualities that are only an advantage in the business world.

Remember the Seventh Commandment of Psychostructure: *I will eliminate (or at least minimize) milk, bread, and alcohol in my diet.*

8. QUESTION AND ANSWER TIME

No matter how well anything is explained, there inevitably remain some questions in the mind of the listener. This chapter consists of questions that are most frequently asked by my patients.

Q: WHAT IS THE USUAL RATE OF WEIGHT LOSS AFTER STARTING THE PROGRAM?

A: A man can expect to lose approximately twenty-one pounds per month. A woman will lose approximately twelve to fifteen pounds per month. These are average figures only. Some patients lose more; some lose less. Just as your body weight fluctuates normally due to variations in diet and exercise from week to week, so also will any intentional or structured weight loss vary between individuals.

Q: WILL CUTTING CALORIES BELOW 700 A DAY SPEED UP THE PROCESS OF LOSING WEIGHT?

A: No. In fact, this can be self-defeating due to the metabolic rate dropping when the intake of food is below 700 calories a day.

Q: I ONCE HAD NO FOOD AT ALL OVER A WEEK-END, AND LOST FIVE POUNDS, SO WHY CAN'T I STARVE TWO DAYS A WEEK AND SPEED UP MY WEIGHT LOSS?

A: No food means no salt. No salt mean rapid water loss by the system. You didn't lose five pounds of fat. You lost five pounds of water space. Believe me, if there were any short cuts, I'd not only know about them, but would prescribe them because I know how anxious you are to lose weight. The quickest and safest way to lose is to stick to my diet: which means 700 calories a day. No more, no less!

Q: IS IT TRUE THAT A KETOGENIC DIET IS THE QUICKEST WAY TO LOSE WEIGHT?

A: No. There is no significant difference in weight loss between ketogenic diets and any other systems, provided the daily calorie consumption is the same.

Q: WHAT IS THE MOST IMPORTANT ITEM IN A DIET?

A: Protein, which is needed for the growth and maintenance of the tissues. To put it simply: protein builds the body, and energy (fat, carbohydrates—calories) makes it function.

Q: THE IDEA OF THREE SMALL MEALS A DAY IS LESS APPEALING THAN ONE LARGE MEAL. CAN'T I CONSUME MY 700 CALORIES AT ONE MEAL?

A: No. Studies have proven that a series of small meals each day enhances weight loss more effectively than one large meal. Our normal eating pattern is three meals a day, which is better for your system, both physically and psychologically.

Q: I HAVE SOME PSYCHOLOGICAL PROBLEMS. SHOULD I TRY TO OVERCOME THESE *BEFORE* ATTEMPTING TO LOSE WEIGHT?

A: No. Many of the hang-ups common among obese people stem from their being overweight. Do not fall into the trap of being advised to clean up your psychological problems before you start dieting. In my experience, I have found that patients with psychological problems tend to become extremely anxious when they seek to understand and solve these problems, and this anxiety makes it very difficult for them to lose weight. Treatment of obesity must go hand-in-hand with treatment of psychological problems.

Q: MY CHILD IS STARTING TO PUT ON WEIGHT. WHAT SHOULD I DO?

A: Eliminate between meal snacks, especially the traditional after-school milk and cookies. Cut down on meal portions, and eliminate milk entirely, with the exception of low-fat or skim milk in small portions. Substitute daily exercise in the yard for that hour of late-afternoon television viewing. Include some of your own low-calorie dishes in your child's diet. (NOTE: See Chapter 8 on milk and milk products.)

Q: I'VE HEARD ACUPUNCTURE WORKS WONDERS WITH OVERWEIGHT. DO YOU RECOMMEND THIS?

A: No. I've known several patients who tried acupuncture to lose weight. All they lost was their money.

Q: WHICH FOODS ARE MOST HARMFUL FOR OBESE PEOPLE?

A: Sugar and carbohydrates, because they stimulate the appetite; also highly concentrated foods such as butter, margarine, and cheese.

Q: YOU SAY EXERCISE IS ESSENTIAL IN YOUR PROGRAM. WHAT IF A PERSON IS SO OVERWEIGHT THAT EXERCISE ISN'T POSSIBLE?

A: I've yet to find an obese person who is unable to move, and exercise is only bodily movement done with varying degrees of effort and in a particular pattern to give all muscles a necessary workout. No matter what a person's size, he can start his daily exercise with a short structured walk, gradually increasing to two miles a day. However, just as I have recommended a thorough physical examination before starting your diet, so also should you check with your doctor about the advisability of exercise. He

155

may suggest you delay starting daily exercise until you have lost a certain amount of weight because of a particular physical problem you may have. Exercise is, nevertheless, essential every day, not only to assist in a permanent weight-loss program but to maintain your system in top physical condition at all times.

Q: IS THE ILEAL BYPASS OPERATION ADVISABLE AS A MEANS OF WEIGHT REDUCTION?

A: The ileal bypass operation is a procedure fraught with great complications, and should be undertaken only after a thorough physical and psychological examination. In my opinion, such drastic measures are advisable only if the obesity is of such magnitude that it totally disables the patient or threatens his life. From a common sense viewpoint, isn't it preferable to follow a proven diet than to indulge in an expensive and hazardous operation?

Q: DO CALORIES REALLY MATTER THAT MUCH?

A: As Cleopatra might have said, you bet your sweet asp! Any doctor, clinic or weight-reduction system that promises permanent control without counting calories can only be concerned with reducing your finances instead of your flab. In most cases, excessive consumption of calories will cause your body to become overweight. Restricting the number of calories you consume at each meal is the only way of ridding yourself of fat, and keeping it off permanently.

Q: WHY DO YOU PRESCRIBE ONLY 700 CALORIES A DAY?

A: I have found 700 calories is the quickest way to bring down body weight and still include all the essential food elements you need for health. You would still lose at 800, or 900 calories, but your rate of weight loss would be slowed down, and once an obese person has decided to do something about losing weight, he usually wants to achieve his goal as quickly as possible.

Q: DOESN'T EXERCISE INCREASE THE APPETITE?

A: No. Exercise reduces the appetite, which is why I recommend taking a brief walk when a patient feels hungry. This tends to decrease any urge to eat more than you should.

Q: WHY IS IT SO MANY AMERICANS SUFFER FROM OVERWEIGHT?

A: Our imaginative inventors have produced an excess of labor-saving devices, from the Model T to remote-control TV, all of which have cut down on our essential physical activity. We have become less active as a nation, and the more we sit, the more we spread. In addition, due to the sophistication of the food industry, there are richer and more fattening foods available which, through aggressive advertising, we are prompted to purchase, making the pantry a conglomeration of high-calorie concoctions instead of a storehouse of staple foods needed only for nutrition.

Q: SHOULD ONE ELIMINATE SALT FROM A DIET IN ORDER TO LOSE WEIGHT?

A: Yes. However, there is no need to avoid salt entirely. Salt substitute should be used, and no salt should be added in cooking food. In reality, *total* elimination of salt from the diet is impossible. Cutting down on added salt, however, will result in more even weight loss. A diet that does not restrict salt will produce an up-and-down pattern of reduction due to the sporadic retention of water in the system. In addition, refraining from salt has a salutary effect on blood pressure.

Q: DO YOU RECOMMEND THE USE OF DIET PILLS?

A: No. Appetite depressants are only a temporary aid in reducing, and the long-term use of potent medications, such as dexedrine, is to be avoided for health reasons and to avoid addiction.

Q: IS IT TRUE TAKING THYROID HELPS ONE TO LOSE WEIGHT?

A: Only if you have a low thyroid function, something your doctor can determine for you. Those with normal glandular activity will not benefit by taking thyroid.

Q: WHAT IS THE GREATEST MISCONCEPTION ABOUT DIETING TODAY?

A: I would say: most obese people regard their previous daily eating routine as normal, and their period of dieting as abnormal. The opposite is the truth: *abnormal* eating habits lead to obesity, while controlling your daily intake of food is *normal*. In other words, to maintain a normal, healthy weight level, an individual prone to obesity *must* regard his daily diet as his normal pattern of eating, not just for that period at the start of my program when large amounts of excess weight are being eliminated, but forever, because reverting to previous eating habits in any way will naturally result in a return of the overweight condition.

Again, this is largely a mental readjustment, which is why psychostructure is so successful. You alter not only your weight, but your mental approach to food. Your basic attitudes are changed, your outlook altered until adherence to a certain number of calories each day becomes automatic, and you regard this restriction on your diet as *normal,* because without it, you would become obese again, which is *abnormal.* In this regard, the 700 calorie maximum is prescribed only for that period during which you bring your weight down to the desired level, after which calories may be increased to 1000, 1500, and more, *provided no weight gain is evidenced under the increased allowance.* But you *must* understand fully that those days of a 3000 to 5000 daily calorie intake are gone forever!

Q: DO YOU RECOMMEND WIRING THE TEETH TOGETHER TO PREVENT EATING AS A MEANS OF LOSING WEIGHT?

A: Definitely not! This is not only dangerous, but it is only a temporary measure, and once the wires are removed, the patient will revert to previous eating habits because he has not changed his attitude towards his problem, which is the key factor in the success of the psychostructure program.

Q: IS WALKING ESSENTIAL, OR CAN I SUBSTITUTE SOME OTHER TYPE OF EXERCISE?

A: *Yes,* walking is essential, and *no,* I do not recommend substituting any other activity for patients able to walk. However, I do welcome a patient who, in *addition* to a daily walk, engages in other exercise, such as tennis or swimming. Walking, when you stop to think about it, can be done almost anytime, anywhere and it doesn't cost you a cent; moreover, once you get into the habit of a daily walk, you will find incredible enjoyment, both physically and psychologically.

Q: I BELIEVE I ONLY EAT TOO MUCH BECAUSE I'M ALWAYS TENSE AND NERVOUS. HOW CAN I HANDLE THESE STRESSES WHICH SEEM TO BE A PART OF MY LIFE?

A: Tensions that result from your particular lifestyle can be worked off by exercise (one of the best methods I know) or, if you prefer, by taking your mind off yourself through conversations with friends (in person or on the phone), playing cards or indulging in needlework, which is equally effective for men and women. It is a sad fact of life that today's hectic pace, especially in our major cities, has led to many psychological problems related to stress; but eating is not the answer! Just as you learn through my program to restructure your attitudes, you must learn to rise above daily pressures and irritations. Many men and women utilize meditation as a means of combatting nervous tension, a philosophy I recommend very highly, because this helps you get your mind back on the right track once more; and the ultimate controlling factor in everything we do is the mind.

Q: IS IT ADVISABLE TO DIET DURING PREGNANCY?

A: Yes, most definitely! A baby will not become malnourished if the mother is on a diet because the fetus is, in actuality, a parasite within the body that draws all its needed nourishment from the system, no matter how much or how little food is ingested by the mother. An obese woman is only doing herself and her unborn child a favor by reducing during pregnancy because the closer you are to your normal weight, the less complications are likely to ensue. Again, this is a matter to be discussed with your doctor, who will naturally be taking care of you at this time.

Q: IS IT ADVISABLE FOR AN OBESE PERSON TO INDULGE IN SEX?

A: If relations are possible and not uncomfortable, yes; in fact, satisfying your biological urges constitutes one of the more enjoyable forms of exercise that can only benefit your weight reduction program! Obese women are physically able to have intercourse though many resist the idea because of embarrassment over their appearance, which is why so many overweight women are sexually frustrated, a condition they satisfy by eating, which only compounds the problem. An obese man will find his sexual performance vastly improved after losing weight for obvious reasons. Bedroom athletics do, after all, require a certain degree of unencumbered pelvic gyrations that can often become exhausting with fifty pounds of excess flab around the waist!

Q: IS PLASTIC SURGERY RECOMMENDED TO REMOVE SAGGING SKIN AFTER COMPLETING A WEIGHT REDUCTION PROGRAM?

A: Yes, especially with individuals who have lost a large amount of weight, such as 100 pounds or more, which can leave an apron of outer flesh hanging in unsightly folds. This unfortunate condition can be minimized by your daily exercise, but for those extreme cases, plastic surgery can help restore a firm covering of skin over the body. The procedures are not without complications, but the results in general are very gratifying. I could recommend, however, that you go to a reputable surgeon well experienced in such an operation. There's a big difference between minor cosmetic surgery and what amounts to a major reconstruction job!

Q: DOES IT HELP TO TAKE HCG SHOTS WHILE ON A DIET?

A: No. Certain chemical therapies can result in weight loss, but often at the risk of dangerous side effects. In addition, the weight inevitably returns when the patient resumes his former eating habits. Psychostructure involves no drugs, and weight loss is permanent.

Q: DOES BEING OBESE LIMIT ONE'S LIFESPAN?
A: Studies indicate that obesity *itself* does not lessen your chances of a long life. However, obesity leads to other health problems that can cause early death, such as heart disease. Come to think of it, I have never seen a really old obese person.

Q: SHOULD I GIVE UP EATING OUT AT RESTAURANTS WHILE ON A DIET?
A: Not as long as you maintain control over your food, and plan your meal before entering a restaurant. *Know* what you will order and don't be tempted to indulge in unstructured eating. Again, let me stress: "being on a diet" must, for permanent control of your weight, refer to the rest of your life, not just to those months during which you reduce your weight to your normal, healthy desired level. Remember, proper eating is a lifetime project!

Q: DO THE HEALTH PROBLEMS CAUSED BY OBESITY DISAPPEAR AFTER RETURNING TO A NORMAL WEIGHT?
A: In most cases, yes. An overweight person with diabetes usually finds his diabetes disappearing along with his obesity. Often high blood pressure returns to normal. Hyperlipidemia (high cholesterol and triglycerides) usually return to normal. You can only become an overall healthier person by losing excess weight.

Q: SHOULD LAXATIVES BE TAKEN WHILE DIETING?
A: No. I recommend stool softeners to my patients who may suffer from constipation during their initial period of weight loss. Laxatives can only deplete the system of potassium, which is essential to your overall health. A good stool softener is Serutan.

Q: ARE VITAMINS NECESSARY WHILE DIETING?
A: Anyone on a very low calorie diet is wise to take a multi-vitamin-mineral capsule each day, to make sure your system is

getting the minimum daily requirements of vitamins and minerals. Check with your doctor or pharmacist for a recommended brand.

Q: YOU SAY YOUR SYSTEM OF DIETING IS FOR LIFE. ISN'T IT DANGEROUS TO CONTINUE DIETING FOR LONG PERIODS OF TIME?

A: No, but it certainly *is* dangerous to remain overweight for long periods. There is no danger in restricting your daily diet provided the protein content is adequate, which it definitely is in the suggested weekly menus included in this book. The body must have protein to rebuild the tissue, whereas your health is only jeopardized by an excessive intake of foods that result in fat.

Q: IS IT TRUE THAT SOME PEOPLE CAN DIET SO LONG THAT THEY LOSE THEIR APPETITE COMPLETELY AND NEVER FEEL LIKE EATING?

A: Yes. Known as *anorexia nervosa,* this condition does occur with some people, though none of my patients have suffered from it as a result of my program. Patients with anorexia nervosa have a tendency not to recognize their condition. If you have a friend or relative who has been dieting and has lost a large amount of weight and still continues to diet so that body weight drops far below normal, you should urge the person to seek medical help.

Q: I HAVE A SLUGGISH METABOLISM. WILL DIETING AND WEIGHT LOSS IMPROVE MY METABOLISM?

A: Many patients on my diet and exercise program find that as their weight begins to fall, their activity level increases, which of course only makes it easier for them to continue losing weight. Although this overall process is related to the metabolic rate, I cannot say whether a person's metabolism is truly affected.

Q: IS IT HARMFUL TO ONE'S SYSTEM TO GO UP AND DOWN THE SCALE, LOSING WEIGHT, GAINING IT BACK, AND THEN LOSING IT ONCE MORE?

A: It's better to have lost and gained than never to have lost at all! I would say that any weight loss, or anything you do to prevent weight gain, is beneficial to the body. Of course, the secret to preventing this up-and-down-the-scale syndrome is to start my program of psychostructure and stick to it until your weight is normal; then gradually you can increase your calories each day from 700 to 1000 or 1500, but *only* after you have accomplished your planned weight reduction, and *only* if there is no increase in weight following the increase in calories; if there is, of course, it's back to 700 per day again! The purpose of any program like mine is to keep your weight at a normal level, week in, week out, for the rest of your life, which is the way it should be.

Q: IS MILK ADVISABLE FOR AN ADULT AS A DAILY PART OF THE DIET?

A: Not if he has a weight problem. There is much good nutrition in milk, but there are also items that are hazardous to weight control: too much sugar, and too much fat. Too many calories, period! If you are accustomed to drinking milk, I suggest you learn to replace this with liquids that have few, if any calories, such as unsugared iced tea or coffee, or any of the many diet soft drinks on the market; and best of all, plain water.

Q: ONCE I ACHIEVE MY DESIRED WEIGHT LEVEL, MAY I EAT ANYTHING I WANT?

A: Absolutely NOT! A person prone to obesity can only control his weight by controlling what he eats. This does not mean your daily diet is dull and boring; as you've seen from the planned menus in this book, there are many dishes that are tasty, tempting and fully satisfying, even with limited amounts. Very obviously, however, fluffy cream pies, and broiled lobster smothered with half a pound of melted butter must be avoided, together with any food that would make you exceed your required maximum calories per meal. The name of the game is counting calories, and if you want to retain your slender shape for the rest of your life, you must accept this fact, and live your life accordingly.

Q: IS IT ESSENTIAL TO START OFF YOUR DIET AT THE STUELKE CLINIC IN DURHAM, NORTH CARO-

LINA, LIKE SOME PEOPLE I KNOW? CAN'T YOU GET THE SAME RESULTS AT HOME?

A: Many patients *do* come to my clinic, but only because their home environment makes it difficult to complete the requirements of my program. Some people find the tensions, distractions and family scene at home incompatible with the dedication required to lose weight; so they take time off, come to my clinic and complete their initial weight loss under the controlled conditions I have set up which make it easier to maintain the daily routine. After losing a desired number of pounds, they return home and continue the program.

This does not mean you can't overcome obesity at home, for all the necessary directives are included in this book; but it does require complete concentration and dedication, and daily watchfulness over every bit of food you eat.

Q: WOULD A DAILY SAUNA OR STEAM BATH HELP ME LOSE WEIGHT?

A: I do *not* recommend saunas or steam baths for losing weight at any time. You might lose weight, but it would be water, not fat, and you would be robbing your body of valuable salts excreted in your sweat.

Q: DOES MASSAGE HELP IN LOSING WEIGHT?

A: Only for the masseur! A massage is a relaxing sensual experience which can calm jangled nerves, but it does nothing to help the body lose weight.

Q: I AM RELUCTANT TO GO ON YOUR DIET BECAUSE EVERY TIME I'VE LOST A FEW POUNDS I START LOOKING HAGGARD AND MORE THAN MIDDLE-AGED. CAN I LOSE WEIGHT WITHOUT STARTING TO LOOK LIKE A STARVING REFUGEE?

A: Many people on a diet complain about their facial appearance at first. This drawn look is caused mostly by dehydration, and can often be overcome by proper intake of fluids. However, this situation occurs only at the start of a major period of dieting.

Once your normal weight level is reached, your face will resume its usual healthy appearance.

Q: WILL LOSING EXCESS WEIGHT RESULT IN MY LOSING MY STRETCH MARKS?

A: No. Weight loss will not eliminate stretch marks, some of which fade in time.

Q: IS THERE ANYTHING YOU CAN DO ABOUT THE HAIR LOSS THAT OCCURS DURING DIETING?

A: Yes. Be sure your protein intake is adequate. Some hair loss is normal, but any hair lost during a period of strict dieting will grow back. Should any hair loss continue, you should check with your doctor as it could be due to a zinc deficiency in your diet, which can naturally be corrected.

Q: THERE ARE SO MANY DIETS AVAILABLE TO-DAY. HOW CAN ONE TELL WHICH ARE ANY GOOD?

A: By checking with your doctor to make sure any diet is adequate, is not a "fad" diet, and that it contains sufficient protein. There are many diets which are based on sound nutritional principles, but remember these are merely "diets"—a means of limiting your daily consumption of fattening foods—in contrast to psychostructure, which enables you to learn the reason behind your obesity, to change your lifestyle, and restructure not only your eating habits, but your mental approach to your problem, which is the most important factor in any plan of weight reduction. Without a change of attitude, any weight loss accomplished through a "diet" will only be temporary. You are concerned with maintaining a normal healthy weight level *permanently*, which involves altering your mental processes as well as your physical appearance. It is no "gimmick!" The psychostructure system is the result of years of research, study, and proven results from thousands of people who have achieved slender, healthy bodies as a result of following my system. You can, too, provided you stick to the rules, and employ patience, perseverance, and dedication. I can show you *how*, but *you* have to do the work, follow through, and reach your goal of a new body and a new outlook on yourself and your health.

Q: I WANT TO LOSE WEIGHT, BUT I HAVE A HUS-BAND AND THREE CHILDREN, NONE OF WHOM ARE OVERWEIGHT. HOW CAN I POSSIBLY FOLLOW YOUR PROGRAM AND STILL COOK THE REGULAR FAMILY MEALS?

A: There is nothing in my diet menu that cannot or should not be eaten by every member of your family. So, how do you cook for them? Simple. Cook your own diet menu, and at mealtimes, dish up the quantity prescribed for you, and serve larger portions for the others at the table. There are more than enough selections to enable you to have an interesting variety of dishes for all meals. If a particular food item is forbidden for you, and someone in your house wants it—well, it's confrontation time! I suggest a compromise in such a case: if one of your children wants pie and ice cream, send them out for it, but with instructions they are not to bring it home, but to eat it elsewhere. (Remember out of sight, out of mind . . .) If your family shares your desire for you to lose weight, they should not object to *giving* a little so you'll ultimately *take* off those extra pounds!

Q: DO YOU REALLY BELIEVE OTHER MEMBERS OF A FAMILY WILL UNDERSTAND AND COOPERATE WHEN SOMEONE DECIDES TO GO ON A DIET?

A: Yes. I believe they can, and they will—but only if you tell them why your new lifestyle is necessary, and why their cooperation is essential to your success. I am quite aware (because I've heard it too many times) that most of us do not regard obesity as a disease, or as a major health problem. We are too used to thinking of people as either thin or fat—two basic types that we happen to be stuck with. All our lives we hear jokes about fat people. We talk about "middle-age spread" as being part of growing older. We laugh at the fat lady at the circus. Through generations of mental preconditioning, the human race has come to accept obesity as being merely a variation in physical form, instead of what it really is: an abnormality caused in most cases by an abnormal eating pattern.

If you have a difficult time soliciting your family's cooperation, ask your doctor to drop in for a family counsel, so he can help explain not only the *reason*, but the *necessity* for your going on a diet and losing weight which might, in time, cause more serious problems and even possibly your early demise. No child will welcome the idea of losing a parent, and no partner in a marriage relishes the idea of being single again because of the early death of the other partner. Despite cynics who might quote the rising divorce statistics, people still do not marry with the idea of breaking up, intentionally or unexpectedly. I may be an old-fashioned romantic, but I believe a man and wife marry for love, hoping that their union will be forever. Families are bound by love; each member cares for the other—and this caring should be the key factor in making everyone appreciate what a fat person faces, and the dangers that exist in going through life grossly overweight. So what if it means a change in the kitchen routine, a change in the amount and type of food stored, a change in the daily menu? When you think about it, this is little enough to ask to help restore one of the family to health again.

Too often resistance to certain aspects of my program stem from over-reaction. "I couldn't possibly do all that," is a statement I've heard many times from my patients. But they *do* it, and wind up slender, healthy and happy—completely happy with themselves for the first time in their lives; then they laugh about the objections they raised before starting my program.

So never use your family as an excuse *not* to lose weight. They'll cooperate, because after you've explained the alternatives, they'll be just as eager for you to diet as you are.

Q: MY DOCTOR HAS SAID MANY TIMES I'LL LOSE WEIGHT IF I CAN ONLY KEEP MY MOUTH CLOSED INSTEAD OF EATING SO MUCH. HOW DO I EXPLAIN TO HIM THAT THIS ISN'T THE PROBLEM?

A: It's not your place to explain anything to a doctor, especially one like yours who obviously does not understand the dynamics and proper treatment of obesity. However, after reading this book and hopefully realizing that your problem is mental as well as physical, share it with your own doctor—and then go forward *together* to start getting your weight down, and keeping it down for the rest of your life: You, your doctor, and psychostructure—that's a combination *guaranteed* to cure your obesity. If this doesn't work, change your doctor!

Q: THE METROPOLITAN LIFE INSURANCE CHART OF DESIRABLE WEIGHTS LISTS DIFFERENT WEIGHTS FOR DIFFERENT FRAMES. DOES THIS REFER TO THE THREE DIFFERENT BODY TYPES YOU TALK ABOUT?

A: No. The three different body types (see page 22) are the three basic body types in the human race. Metropolitan lists "frames" because we have, over the years, come to regard large people as having a large "frame," small people as having a small "frame," which has a bearing upon your suitable weight; in actuality, however, there is no such thing as a small, medium, or large frame because if you weigh the skeletons of all types of people of the same height, you will find very little difference. (Someone you might consider having a "large frame" is more likely a small or medium frame individual who is overweight!) No person's bones are any bigger than the next, with two exceptions: members of the black races, who are endowed with a heavier muscle structure, making the ideal weight listing a little low for them; and football players and weight lifters whose bodies are heavily muscled, thereby invalidating the ideal weight listed on the chart. However, for the average man or woman, the ideal weight listings are accurate enough.

Q: WHAT EXACTLY IS MEANT BY "IDEAL" WEIGHT?

A: Ideal weight refers to the number of pounds at which you will live the longest. I also consider ideal weight as the weight at which you look your best.

Here is the listing of desirable weights that I follow, listing the average weights for men and women age twenty-five and over, from five feet two inches through six feet four inches.

DESIRABLE WEIGHTS
(± 10%)

Men of Ages 25 and Over			Women of Ages 25 and Over		
Height		*Average*	*Height*		*Average*
Feet	Inches		Feet	Inches	
5	2	124	4	10	102
5	3	127	4	11	104
5	4	130	5	0	107
5	5	133	5	1	110
5	6	137	5	2	113
5	7	141	5	3	116
5	8	145	5	4	120
5	9	149	5	5	123
5	10	153	5	6	128
5	11	158	5	7	132
6	0	162	5	8	136
6	1	167	5	9	140
6	2	171	5	10	144
6	3	176	5	11	148
6	4	181	6	0	152

(Courtesy of the Metropolitan Life Insurance Company)

Q: IS THE METROPOLITAN LIFE INSURANCE CHART OF IDEAL WEIGHTS TO BE TAKEN AS ABSOLUTE?

A: The chart applies to most people, but there are some exceptions. For example, there are those whose station in life and lifestyle affect their ideal weight. A grandmother with fourteen grandchildren who is five foot two inches would be perfectly normal at 120 pounds, but her glamorous grand-daughter who is also five foot two inches and a fashion model would be considered overweight at 120 pounds.

Q: IF ONE IS A FEW POUNDS OVER THE IDEAL WEIGHT LISTED ON THE METROPOLITAN CHART, SHOULD ONE BE CONSIDERED OVERWEIGHT?

A: No. You can add or subtract ten percent and you would still fall into the range which I consider healthy. In regard to obesity, I consider the terms "healthy" and "normal" or "ideal" as synonymous, because being more than ten percent over your ideal weight is unhealthy, just as any obese condition is unhealthy.

Q: IS THERE A WAY OF ASSESSING ONE'S IDEAL WEIGHT WITHOUT REFERRING TO A CHART?

A: Yes. If you are a person who did not become obese until adulthood, you could consider your weight at age seventeen as being a good, ideal weight for you. For those who have had a weight problem since childhood, this rule-of-thumb does not apply, naturally.

Q: DOESN'T THE BODY WEIGHT DIMINISH NORMALLY AS WE GROW OLDER?

A: Yes. At age seventeen, a person five foot two inches and weighing 113 pounds would be an ideal weight, but at age sixty, this same person would be overweight at 113 pounds. Roughly, the ideal weight drops one pound for every five years of life. A person weighing 120 at age twenty should thereby weigh 110 at age seventy.

Q: ISN'T 'MIDDLE-AGE' SPREAD INEVITABLE?

A: No. This unhappy condition may come to many of us, but is not natural. Proper diet and exercise can keep your waistline just as trim at fifty as it was at twenty. In addition, the muscle mass in the human body slowly but inevitably diminishes with age.

Q: WHAT'S A GOOD EASY WAY TO TELL IF YOU'RE OVERWEIGHT?

A: There are two ways: the pinch test and the twist test. The first: pinch your flesh between thumb and forefinger, preferably between your ribcage and hips. If, after gripping your skin, your thumb and forefinger are more than one-half inch apart, you're obese! If you're unable to pinch more than a smidgeon of skin, consider yourself in good shape. Second: for the twist test, stand unclothed in front of the mirror and twist your shoulders to the right and then to the left. If your stomach fails to turn with your shoulders, but is delayed in its movement, you've got a problem! In my years of treating obesity, I have accumulated other little indications of present or imminent obesity, such as: people with a weight problem tend to steer clear of mirrors and shop windows. (That tell-tale midriff bulge is sometimes too hard to take!); heavier men and women lean more to wearing loafers than lace-up shoes. (Have you tried tying a shoelace while reaching over a distended belly?) When sitting down obese people spread their legs instead of crossing them.

Q: ISN'T A PLUMP BABY HEALTHIER THAN A THIN BABY?

A: Definitely *not*! Fat children are not healthy, no matter what doting grandmothers will say to the contrary. Traditionally, skinny kids are regarded with disdain, and derogatory remarks are often levelled at the mother for neglecting her baby. The truth is: a skinny boy or girl will talk sooner, walk sooner and have a faster intellectual development, as well as being easier to toilet train, than a fat baby. The body develops better slightly underweight than overweight.

Q: WHAT IS THE MORE IMPORTANT FACTOR IN A CHILD BECOMING OBESE: GENETIC FACTORS OR DIET AFTER BIRTH?

A: There may be a genetic predisposition to body types, but heredity is very insignificant compared with the social and environmental influences after birth. If the parents overeat, their child will be similarly inclined. If food is important to parents, it will also assume importance to the child.

Q: DOES OBESITY IN CHILDHOOD AFFECT A YOUNGSTER'S RATE OF MATURITY?

A: Very often obesity prior to and during puberty can be a serious detriment to a child's sexual-social development. While the biological maturation occurs, the important psychological advancement is hampered. As I have illustrated, obesity is an unhealthy condition, both physically and mentally. It is not uncommon to see formerly obese males of thirty exhibiting the same approach to the opposite sex as a fourteen year old after losing weight. It is a rather tragic phenomenon to see a thirty year old man trying to make up for fifteen lost years!

Q: DOES OBESITY AFFECT A WOMAN'S SEXUALITY?

A: Obesity is not a deterrent nor a detriment to sexual development and potential activity in the female. In the male, however, obesity is a definite complication, both psychologically and physically, to the proper and complete fulfillment of the sex act.

Q: AS A BUSINESSMAN, I CLOSE MOST OF MY DEALS OVER LUNCH. HOW CAN I POSSIBLY ADHERE TO MY DIET WHEN TAKING A CLIENT OUT TO A GOURMET RESTAURANT?

A: The ideal solution: do not discuss business over meals! Meet with your associates in your office, complete your negotiations and *then* go on to a restaurant for your meal. If this is impossible for one reason or another, and you feel your financial future will be in jeopardy if you break tradition, follow these simple rules:

First: plan where you will go. Call ahead and ask the restaurant if they can prepare you a meal that coincides with your dietary limitations. Better still, find yourself a good eating place where you can take your clients regularly, and arrange for a regular luncheon for yourself that will not exceed your 150 calories. On arrival, while your client is thumbing through the menu, you can, with great aplomb, greet the waiter and say, "I'll have my usual!" In this way, you will eliminate the possible trauma of explaining to the waiter why you only want a few shrimp and a salad instead of the calorie-laden dishes on the menu.

Second: on your arrival in the restaurant, do not look at the menu. If you do, you'll be lost! It is virtually impossible for a person with a weight problem, who is externally oriented the way we all are, to order a diet meal after looking at the menu.

Third: Get yourself a 3 x 5 file card, and write down in advance what you intend ordering for lunch. Hand this to the waiter, and then forget about food for the moment, especially if your client is still in the process of ordering. People like us who are externally oriented are often influenced by what others order, and many times, at the last minute, despite admirable resolve, you hear your lunch partner order macaroni and cheese, and you switch your fruit plate to the same as his. Result: disaster! Write down in advance what you will order, hand it to the waiter and stick to it!

Remember these three rules: (1) Set up a diet meal in advance with the restaurant, if possible; (2) Do not look at the menu when you sit down; and (3) Write down your intended meal on a card for the waiter.

Q: I FEEL EMBARRASSED DURING A CLIENT LUNCHEON WHEN I REFUSE ALCOHOL. IS THERE ANY WAY TO GET AROUND THIS?

A: Yes. If your client insists on buying you a drink, smile apologetically and explain that you may not drink for three days because you are having a liver function test and your doctor has taken you off alcohol for three days! Most people accept this rational explanation without question, whereas your denial of a drink because of dieting will very often rate a laugh and a jocular insistence that "one drink won't hurt" (and that one drink always leads to another, and another . . . and it's disaster time again!)

Q: MAY I HAVE ONE SMALL DESSERT TO KEEP MY CLIENT COMPANY DURING A BUSINESS LUNCH?

A: *NO!* No desserts! You have to keep your calorie intake below 150. If you order a shrimp cocktail (without sauce) and a plain salad, you'll have a respectable looking plateful when you combine the two and nibble slowly while your client consumes his choice. If you are questioned why you do not have mayonnaise on your salad, blame your doctor again! The same applies to desserts. Remember, following these rules, and at the rate of two business luncheons a week, you'll save yourself 1500 calories a lunch, adding up to about forty pounds a year. Another plus-factor of eating light at lunch: if you consume a 1500 calorie meal for lunch, your mental processes will be slowed down afterwards as the stomach draws blood from other parts of the body (including the brain!) to start the digestive process. So if you eat a light lunch, without alcohol, you'll wind up more alert for that after-lunch business meeting, while your client will be sluggish in comparison.

The above advice regarding business luncheons applies equally well to any type of lunch you may attend with friends, bridge club members, etc. Eating the noon meal in congenial company (business or otherwise) is no excuse to go on an eating binge.

Q: CAN I TAKE A DRINK WHILE ON A DIET?
A: Yes, you *can*. But *may* you? *NO!* (See Chapter 7.)

Q: CAN I DO ANY EXERCISE I PREFER INSTEAD OF THE DAILY TWO MILE WALK YOU PRESCRIBE?
A: If you are so grossly overweight that walking has become almost impossible, you will naturally have to wait until you get down to that weight where you *can* walk. If there are some calisthenics you are able to do, fine. Any exercise is good, and your doctor can advise you on this matter, even provide you with suggested routines you might be able to do. But whatever exercise you undertake, nothing is as good or as effective at helping you lose weight than a daily two-mile walk. This is a *fact*.

Remember the Eighth Commandment of Psychostructure: *I will clean my mental house and follow every rule to successfully restructure my lifestyle.*

9. YOU ARE NOT ALONE

Patients who come to my clinic in Durham not only have the advantage of a controlled environment in which to start their weight-loss program, but they gain comfort and renewed determination from being able to share their experiences with other patients in the group sessions that are part of the program. Meeting and hearing about everyone's problems creates a team effect, a joint battle against overweight, which in turn reinforces individual effort. Patients agree they gain a great deal by telling their stories and hearing how others are losing weight day by day.

Obviously this type of benefit is impossible for those of you at home, which is the reason for this chapter. I am including a selection of case histories from my files, documented examples of men and women of all ages who have successfully lost weight through psychostructure and who are continuing to maintain a normal healthy weight level.

Naturally, names have been changed, but the facts are there to give additional impetus to your own efforts as you begin your own program. By reading how others have overcome their obesity, you will realize that no situation is hopeless provided you approach your problem positively, follow every prescribed step, and maintain an unwavering belief in your ultimate success.

Case History #1: John P.

John P. works as a highly paid executive in one of the largest corporations in the world. His daily routine is long, critical, and results in never-ending deadlines and crises, all of which contribute to John being under constant pressure and stress. Apart from his office duties, John is required to attend frequent business luncheons, banquets, dinners, and participate in a great deal of client entertaining, all of which led to more than mere middle-age spread.

When John came to me, he was grossly overweight due to overindulgence in rich foods, together with unscheduled snacking, and nervous eating in between meals. Because of the demands of his job, he anticipated an above-average difficulty in completing my program; yet he did. He lost weight and has continued to maintain a normal body weight ever since.

John succeeded because he adhered to my program, down to the minutest detail. In his work, he was successful because he applied himself to proven principles of business management, and he approached my program in the same manner: he knew psycho-structure was a proven method of weight control, and he followed the system every step of the way.

He exhibited a total dedication to losing weight, just as he is totally dedicated to his work. Accustomed to organizing business strategies to cover every eventuality, he began reorganizing his lifestyle, restructuring his environment, and reprogramming his own attitudes and responses.

Now, at any of the business luncheons or dinners he attends, John does not fall victim to the temptations of the menu. He knows precisely what his meal will include, and he orders only those foods which are on his diet, thereby maintaining his daily caloric allowance.

Accustomed in business to having his orders carried out, John insists upon absolute adherence to the type and quantity of food he orders. If he decides on a six ounce steak, medium rare, with half a baked potato and a small salad with vinegar or lemon juice, that is all he will accept from the waiter. He has learned not to be tempted by tantalizing smells from the kitchen; nor is he intimidated by persistent well-meaning waiters and friends. He has learned, happily, that to maintain his slender build, he has to continue following the dietary limitations that enabled him to lose weight in the first place.

His secret is absolute structure and planning, plus a strong, assertive command of any situation affecting what he eats. He is not relying on will power (which so often weakens) but on *intellectual control* to maintain the daily routine essential to keeping his weight at the desired level. His *mind* is in control of his *body,* which is as it should be in psychostructure.

I am especially pleased with John's success in overcoming obesity because he proves that anyone high up the executive ladder, with almost intolerable pressures and demands on his time, can complete my program and restructure his lifestyle to coincide with a prescribed pattern for preventing the body from becoming overweight.

Case History #2: Theresa W.

Theresa is now an attractive, slender seventeen-year-old young woman, active and interested in life with a host of friends and no shortage of dates; but when I first met her she was a grossly overweight teenager with little about her that could be called appealing, including her manner, which was surly, withdrawn, and blatantly antagonistic.

Her father, who brought her to me for treatment, confessed that as a baby, Theresa had been chubby, and was, as a result, given the nickname of "Dumpling." Whether the child decided to live up to her nickname or not, I cannot say, but the fact remained that Theresa grew from a chubby baby into a pudgy child who passed into puberty seventy pounds overweight. Her father said she would go through long periods of withdrawal, childishly insisting on having her own way, and sulking if she didn't get it; she became a serious problem for her family.

After several unsuccessful attempts to get Theresa to lose weight, she was brought to my clinic. After a series of conversations with her, I got the impression that she looked upon her stay as merely a means of getting her away from home to avoid embarrassment to her family. She threw frequent temper tantrums, and was extremely anti-social. She obviously hated herself and everyone else included, and rather understandably; she made a rather pathetic sight as she would make her way awkwardly around the building.

Slowly, however, as her weight began falling, she started to respond. She began taking an interest in herself and in other people. She completed her daily exercise routines, and stuck to the structured diet. She began participating in the social programs at the clinic, emerging gradually from her cocoon of fat, and becoming a human being.

By the time she had lost seventy pounds, she was a totally different young woman: active, bubbling with energy and enthusiasm. I found it hard to believe she was the same person who had grudgingly come to my clinic a few months before. She took an interest in her clothes, was concerned over her makeup and hairstyle, and began making plans for her future. On the day she left, she gave me a radiant smile and tremulously murmured her appreciation; her father was even more grateful. "I brought you a hateful, fat kid," he told me, "and you gave me back a healthy, slender daughter."

Theresa still maintains a structured diet each day, and gets her daily exercise; but she follows her program enthusiastically because she has proven to herself how enjoyable life can be without the burden of an obese body to limit her activities and warp her outlook.

Case History #3: Annette M.

So often patients come to me with psychological as well as physical problems, and after delving into their backgrounds, I find their overweight conditions stem directly from emotional conflicts in their lives. Too many of us, embroiled in a family situation, give vent to our frustrations at the dinner table, gaining satisfaction from eating what is denied us in other areas.

Such a case was Annette M., a thirty-five-year-old school teacher who was literally driven to obesity by the effect of a domineering and uncaring mother.

Her father had died when Annette had just started her career, and when her mother suggested that Annette move back home again, she willingly complied, realizing that her mother needed company. From this situation, there grew a very unhealthy dependency between mother and daughter.

Mrs. M. played upon Annette's naturally submissive nature and literally dominated her daughter's life. Annette went nowhere without her mother, who made it her business to make sure she was never alone. She refused to accept the idea of Annette driving "because it was too dangerous to drive in the city." Similarly, she did not want Annette going out at night on the bus or in a taxi for fear of being mugged. Annette's life deteriorated into a dull routine of going to work, then coming home and spending the rest of the day and each evening at home with her mother, who doted on her daughter, preparing delectable meals "much better than that terrible restaurant food" as an added inducement to keep Annette at home. Frustrated and unable to cultivate a life of her own (a boyfriend would have been unthinkable!), Annette turned to food as a substitute satisfaction. She began putting on weight, which slowly eroded what was left of her self-confidence and self-image. On a few occasions, she desperately attempted a diet, would reduce until she was once more presentable, but thanks to her routine and her ever-present mother's cooking, she quickly regained the weight. She found herself becoming more and more enmeshed in her mother's neurotic need for her.

Finally, she gathered what was left of her courage and came to my clinic to take the psychostructure program. As happens with most of my patients, Annette lost not only her obesity, but her lack of self-confidence as well. She lost over sixty pounds, and literally blossomed into a highly attractive woman who was able to spark the remains of her assertiveness, regain a sense of independence, and, at my suggestion, carve her own niche in life away from her mother.

She got herself an apartment, learned to drive, bought a car, and began to develop a circle of friends. Through our counseling and group sessions at the clinic, Annette was able to pinpoint the *cause* of her obesity, and take the necessary steps to prevent a repetition of the circumstances that led to her becoming overweight.

Annette's case is significant in that it illustrates the close relationship between the physical and the psychological aspects of obesity. In most cases, psychological problems are compounded by being overweight, but in Annette's case, her overeating stemmed directly from the frustrations and unnatural lifestyle imposed on her by her mother. (There *are* those who have a vested interest in keeping people fat!) Annette ultimately realized that she had her own life to lead, as she is leading it this very day, slender, attractive, and full of energy, thanks to psychostructure.

Case History #4: Wanda G.

Each of my patients has his or her peculiarities that affect their progress under my program. Some sail through effortlessly, but others tend to balk at certain of the restrictions and rules. Wanda G. was an example of the latter case, which I am citing to illustrate the necessity to follow *every single* procedure spelled out in psychostructure.

Wanda is a very intelligent businesswoman who entered my program to lose a desired forty pounds. During the first few weeks she was at the clinic, Wanda expressed a certain cynicism over some parts of the program, especially when her weight loss was uneven.

She would lose four pounds during the week, go off for the weekend and come back on Monday, having regained four pounds and often more! I realized that she obviously went on an eating binge during her weekends, so I insisted she document everything she ate. Perhaps her high degree of intelligence gave her the idea she knew more than I did; I cannot say. But she did resist my demands, until after another month went by and her weight had not diminished perceptibly. Finally she relented, and agreed to list everything she ate, down to the last morsel. The results were amazing, and proved that in her case, documentation was the tool she needed to forge the successful conquest of her condition. Faced with the negative reinforcement inherent in writing down every bit of unstructured food consumed, she began eating less, and adhering only to her structured diet. Her weekends were no longer a problem, and dramatically she began losing weight steadily until she achieved her desired level.

Today, she carries our program diary in her purse. For her, documentation is the safeguard against any possible unstructured eating.

Case History #5: Ava S.

I am including this case as an illustration of the vital importance of walking as a daily exercise to help weight control.

Ada and Ava are identical twins in their middle forties. Both are five feet two inches tall; both are unmarried. They live together—two legendary Southern spinsters!

When Ava came to me, she was considerably overweight; yet her sister (her identical twin) was slim. I interviewed them both at the same time and discovered that while they claimed to eat the same food each day, down to the last late-night snack before bed, their work habits were different.

Ada worked as a keypunch operator and walked to work each

day. Ava was a librarian and drove her car to the library because it was too far to walk. How far? A little over a mile, she told me.

I suggested that Ava's weight gain was caused by her lack of exercise, and advised that she, like her sister, walk to work, thereby giving her the two mile minimum walk I prescribe for my patients. The results were predictable: after a short stay at my clinic, Ava's weight dropped to within a few ounces of her sister's, and thereafter and ever since, it has been almost impossible to tell them apart. She has maintained her weight level merely by walking to work each day. This case serves to underline the importance of that two-mile daily walk! Exercise was all that was necessary for Ava's system to maintain a normal weight level.

Case History #6: Emma R.

Emma R. is a woman in her early thirties who, until fairly recently, weighed over 300 pounds. She had, for years, tried one diet after another, losing, then gaining back, until she became desperate and decided to undergo the ileal bypass operation. She knew of the potential problems, but she felt drastic measures were necessary to cope with her excessive obesity.

She entered the hospital, and before the operation, she had the opportunity to speak with several patients who had already undergone the operation. In addition to hearing some unpleasant facts she hadn't expected, Emma heard someone speak about the Stuelke Clinic in Durham, and how successful the psychostructure program is.

By now Emma was more than hesitant about undergoing the bypass operation. She left the hospital and came to my clinic.

She has lost over 100 pounds already, and is thankful at being saved the dubious benefits of the bypass operation. She is still at the clinic, and by the time this book is published, I fully anticipate Emma will be back in society again, slender, healthy and able to enjoy life unhampered by the limitations that often result from having most of the intestines put out of commission.

Case History #7: Clara G. and Martha M.

I have included these two women in the same case history to be able to illustrate the importance of *attitude* in losing weight.

Clara and Martha entered my clinic about the same time. They are both in their early fifties, and at the time they started my program, they both weighed approximately the same. Clara seemed to be a trifle more neurotic than Martha, who appeared to be the stereotype of the fat, jolly lady. Physically, however, they were not dissimilar.

To date, they have each lost a little over sixty pounds, and still have another sixty to lose before reaching their desirable weight level. Despite their progress, Clara remains dissatisfied and frustrated, eager only for the day when she will have lost *all* her excess weight. Martha is frankly overjoyed with her weight loss, and has become even jollier than before, exhibiting a new awareness of life, and exuding an obvious self-confidence in herself. She has taken up some active sports and in addition to her daily walk, she plays tennis three times a week.

Clara, on the other hand, still shuns social contact, and mopes alone, neurotically castigating herself because she hasn't lost more weight, and looking upon her ultimate goal as being almost impossible, despite the fact that she *is* losing weight steadily.

However, and this is the significant punchline: Martha has begun losing *more* each week than Clara. I suspect Martha will achieve her desired total weight loss weeks ahead of Clara. Why? Because she is displaying a *positive* attitude toward not only her program, but to her life in general. She has "rejoined the human race" even though she still has to lose more weight. Clara still looks upon herself as an obese outcast.

I stress again: do not think about your ultimate desired total weight loss. Take each day, each week at a time, and set yourself goals along the way. Such an attitude is essential, as you can see from Clara's case.

Case History #8: Jerry M.

Jerry M. remains one of the most dramatic successes of psychostructure, and living proof that no matter how obese one may be, no condition is hopeless.

When Jerry M. was brought (literally!) into my clinic, he weighed 408 pounds; and for a twenty-four-year-old male, this is tragic. He was not living, but merely existing. He was supported by his family, and indulged in no activity of any kind. No hobbies. No interests. His waking hours were spent sprawled in the living-room, watching television, a routine broken only by visits to the bathroom, the dining room for meals (*massive* meals!), and of course, to his bedroom at night, where he slept on a specially reinforced king size bed. Each morning he had to be helped to his feet. He had nothing to look forward to except dying, which he obviously was doing slowly as his body bloated and deteriorated from inactivity.

His one redeeming feature: he had a sharp, receptive mind, which quickly began understanding the daily routine he would have to follow. He received intense counseling and help every step of the way, and in time, successfully lost *210 pounds!*

He has returned home, continued his daily diet and exercise, and maintained his weight level. The last time we talked, Jerry told me enthusiastically that he really felt as though he had been born again, and that he had only now started living.

Case History #9: Vera T.

Vera T. is another patient of whom I am particularly proud, and another example to reinforce my assertion that *no* case is hopeless. I stress this point because there are many grossly overweight men and women in the world who have reconciled themselves to living their lives as grotesque outcasts and this is ridiculous. If a body has put on weight, it can also lose it, no matter how much.

Vera was twenty-six years of age when she came to my clinic some years ago. She had three children, whom she had placed with her parents while she came to me for treatment. She expected being at the clinic for a long time, because she tipped the scale at 387 pounds.

She applied herself and lost over 200 pounds. She underwent extensive plastic surgery to tighten up her abdomen, and left my clinic, overjoyed at her accomplishment, and fully determined to continue her daily diet restriction and her exercise.

When last we talked, she was continuing to lose, and felt confident she would reach her desired weight level very soon. She is working for the first time in years, and has begun a busy new social life. She admitted she never expected to lose as much as she has, and regards her transformation as a miracle.

To a Bible student, a miracle is a physical manifestation of faith, but I do recall that the good book tells us to "put our shoulder to the wheel." Faith needs action on our part, and I believe for an obese person, a desired weight loss can only result from faith in our innate ability to succeed.

Case History #10: Glenn H.

The importance of one's mental attitudes towards obesity were a pivotal factor in my treatment of Glenn H.—a single man in his early forties who came to me after years of futile attempts to lose weight permanently. Glenn had tried several different diets with temporary success; he went to a doctor who gave him shots that dropped his weight drastically (with some unpleasant side effects, I might add), but always, those extra pounds crept back on his frame, and he became progressively more depressed and frustrated over his obese condition, something he had not always had.

Glenn told me that when he was thirty-seven, his father died, and his semi-invalid mother came to live with Glenn. Although there was another brother in the family with whom she could have stayed, Mrs. H. opted for her youngest and, she said, her favorite son. She failed to realize that Glenn was struggling to get his home improvement business on its feet and was really in less than an ideal position to have her living with him; but he acceded to her wishes nevertheless.

Glenn's already hectic schedule was complicated now by having to rush home in the evening to prepare the dinner and get his mother comfortable. He confessed to being worried continuously over her welfare, and his business began to suffer as a result. Inevitably, Glenn's frustrations had their effect on his eating habits, and he started putting on weight from what he termed "his nervous nibbling" all day and late at night. From a trim 185 he went up to 257 in less than a year. This extra weight brought on back problems, and finally, one night he suffered a ruptured disc and had to be operated upon, yet another psychological burden for him to contend with. Subconsciously, he blamed his mother for his misfortune, yet his devotion to her precluded his taking any action in the matter.

When he finally came to my clinic at his doctor's suggestion, he spilled out this story to my sympathetic ear, and in addition to putting him on the program, I counseled him regarding his personal situation with his mother: I suggested that she remain with his brother, where she was staying during the time Glenn was at my clinic; obviously her presence in his home was a key factor to his problems. Rather reluctantly, he agreed, and after losing forty pounds, he returned home and continued my diet and exercise program. He finally reduced his weight back to 190, where it has remained ever since, just as his mother continued to remain at his brother's house where she received far better care and became happily reconciled to living there with her other son and his wife.

Although Glenn still adheres to a restricted diet, and now he is no longer plagued by the urge to "nibble" as he used to, and his nerves are no longer a problem. He exercises daily, and finds his life once more enjoyable without having to carry round those excess pounds in his body. Mentally, too, his attitudes are more positive and he is able to apply himself to his business without the constant worry of his mother's welfare. He knows she is far better off with his brother, just as he is far better off without having to worry about taking care of her day and night. Today, with the right mental attitude, he is able to lead a fulfilling life and guard himself against any repetition of his obesity.

Case History #11: Clyde and Sarah S.

It is not uncommon to have a husband and wife who both suffer from obesity. Such a case was Clyde and Sarah S., who came to me some years ago with a combined weight of 491 pounds! Since they were both medium height (Clyde five foot nine inches, Sarah five foot six inches) this constituted a gross amount of overweight. I learned they had both been normal weight when they married five years before, but following the sad news that Sarah was unable to have children, they began, without realizing it, seeking substitute satisfactions in food. They joined a wine taster's club and a gourmet cooking class, and while they confessed to "having a ball" at their weekly meetings, they slowly but surely found their weight increasing until Clyde went from 156 to 246, and Sarah ballooned from 130 to 245. They said, jokingly, that their togetherness was so intense that they even weighed the same, which may have some humor lurking someplace, but for me, there was nothing funny about their condition. Obviously they felt the joke had gone far enough, too, for they came to my clinic for a period of treatment, by which time even the dubious delights of their gourmet club had palled. Clyde confessed to me privately that while they still got along famously, their sex life had deteriorated to the point that it had become almost non-existent. He said Sarah was still more than cooperative, but his own obesity made intimacy rather awkward, as well as psychologically inhibiting.

They both made up their minds to stay at the clinic until they had regained their former weight levels. I must say their dedication was admirable. They stayed on their structured diets and indulged in more than merely the two-mile walk daily; they played tennis and swam, and very soon the transformation began taking place.

Three months after they walked into my establishment in Durham, Clyde and Sarah left. Clyde weighed 160 and Sarah was down to 143. Checking with me later, they told me they had dropped even more, and were sticking to their regimen at home, watching every morsel they ate and maintaining their daily exercise routine. Needless to say, the wine tasting and the gourmet club were things of the past. And happily their sex lives had resumed a satisfying frequency once more.

Just as they had become obese together, so also did they lick their problem together, and through mutual self-help, are today maintaining their bodies at the ideal weight level. Sarah's childless condition is no longer a matter of concern to them, either, as they have adopted two children and are now a slender, very happy family of four.

Case History #12: Emily R.

Emily R. is, today, what she was two years ago—a trim, energetic talent agent in New York City who bustles around the Big Apple placing her many clients in films and television commercials; but in 1974, she found that the endless round of business luncheons, dinners, and cocktail parties were slowly but surely adding a pound or two every week, a situation she chose to ignore at the time because she could not afford to say "no" to these gatherings. Her social life was so closely interwoven with her business dealings that she felt if she refused, she might prejudice the consummation of a deal; so Emily drank, ate, and continued her hectic pace, oblivious to her spreading waistline—until one day, a top New York producer referred to her as "that fat broad." Only then did Emily stop to take a good look at herself, and what she saw threw her into a complete state of shock. She had gone from 118 pounds to 156! For a woman like Emily, whose appearance is half the battle to getting into producers' offices, this was like the end of the world!

She had heard about my clinic in Durham, and she took time off from her agency to come down for treatment. She confessed that she was quite aware *why* she had gained weight—it was all those drinks, all that high-calorie food—she saw no way out of her dilemma. To her, this routine was part of her job, and she told me bluntly that she intended to lose forty pounds, but anticipated it coming back as soon as she returned to work.

I told Emily that she would, in fact, lost forty pounds (she proved to be an ideal patient, following every rule to the letter) and stressed my technique for businessmen or women to avoid the very trap into which she had fallen: she had to learn to say "no" as well as to substitute a low-calorie drink for that scotch or martini, and to plan her menu before going to a restaurant with a client. At first Emily was dubious, but she felt it was worth a try. She felt even more positive about my rules after she completed a course of treatment and regained her normal weight again. She returned to New York, slender and bubbling with enthusiasm.

She called me a month later, even more enthusiastic than when she left Durham. She had found no social disgrace in abstaining from alcohol, nor were her luncheons and dinners with clients a disaster because she ordered a diet menu. She was able to conduct her business just as before, but without the ensuing weight problems, simply because she had learned to monitor her drinks and the dishes she ate, thereby keeping her daily intake within acceptable limits and keeping her figure in perfect shape.

As I have stressed over and over again, business parties, luncheons and dinners need not be avoided once you master the secret of how to order and what to drink.

For those of you who might balk at this part of my program, let me emphasize: drinking and eating is an accepted form of social intercourse. It is the getting together, the sharing of company and its pleasures, that make the bar and the restaurant such popular places for social and business activity; but, believe me, it is not the contents of that glass, nor what is on that plate, which determines the success of your get-together. It is your own personality, manner, and speech which add up to being liked and enjoyed; so why feel you have to have alcohol, or a high-calorie meal, in order to insure a successful meeting? Your business deal will be consummated just as well if you are drinking low-cal soda water or eating a plain tossed salad. This isn't theory: it's a proven fact, and part of the proven methods I use in assuring my patients' success in permanently being able to control their obesity.

As you have probably realized, the preceding case histories are all of individuals who have come to my clinic for treatment. Does this mean your results at home will not be as effective? Not at all.

Any patient who requires constant supervision from others could well revert to old bad habits when left alone; which is why the goal of my program, both at my clinic and for you at home, is a totally restructured lifestyle, forever free from obesity. Such an achievement *does* require daily supervision, but to be permanently effective, such supervision *must* come from yourself. As I said before, I can show you *how* to lose weight permanently, but *you* have to do the work!

Psychostructure, in reality, is not just "a diet." To be technically accurate, psychostructure is a total self-rehabilitation program that will not only take off excess weight, but which will restore you to your normal weight level and thereafter enable you to maintain that level through following a new lifestyle that precludes those foods you must avoid and which includes a pattern of behavior essential to your health . . . a pattern you learn to follow instinctively.

There are some cynics who will say all we are talking about is diet and exercise. Sure. There is no other way to maintain a desired body weight all your life. Where psychostructure succeeds is in the restructuring of your attitudes—your mental responses—so that eating right and exercising become an automatic daily activity instead of a regimen you grudgingly follow for a few months in order to bring your weight down.

On my program, we prepare each patient for this role of self-supervision through a series of group sessions. Failures and accomplishments are discussed openly—*honestly*—and through self-analysis, the individual learns how to cope with his own particular problems that have caused his obesity.

While group therapy has proved invaluable in this respect, you can do the same for yourself at home by diligent self-examination and an honest appraisal of your shortcomings. You may wish to form your own club for regular get-togethers with other dieters for mutual morale-building and discussion. Admit to yourself those areas of your life that need changing, and then follow the three cardinal principles: *documentation, exercise,* and *structure,* without which permanent control of your obesity is virtually impossible.

Are there those who say they couldn't possibly do it? I've heard that remark before, and this is normal with some people because this negative response stems from your prior pre-conditioning. The life they have been leading for the past twenty or thirty years has programmed their mind to accept certain daily activities, and any projected change in those activities can cause a negative reaction.

Let me use the following analogy to make my point: from early childhood we are told to brush our teeth morning and night, or preferably after every meal when possible. We grow up with this idea in mind. Our teeth should be brushed every single day. Occasionally we may slip, and go to bed without brushing, but for the most part, every man and woman in the civilized world knows that teeth are to be brushed daily to prevent decay and possible early loss of an essential part of our bodies. Do we, as adults, quibble with this regimen? No. We have realized over the years that it is essential to our well-being and our health. Oral hygiene has become *automatic* and *instinctive.*

The same response and mental attitude has to be cultivated by an obesity-prone person in regard to his daily diet and activities. How? By following a program that guarantees results and which has been proven: PSYCHOSTRUCTURE.

Naturally, this takes time. Any new habit pattern does not occur overnight. You have to persevere, to watch yourself every second, to monitor yourself consciously until your mind becomes impressed with your new pattern of behavior and the regimen thereafter becomes *automatic* and *instinctive,* at which point the possible resistance you exhibit at the start will disappear.

Your success in restructuring your lifestyle is directly related to your degree of desire to overcome your obesity. If you genuinely want to lose weight and maintain a normal healthy level all your life, you'll have no difficulty in following my program and *following it every step of the way*! Thousands of others have done it. You can, too!

To refresh your memory, I am repeating my three steps in detail to stress their importance:

First, *documentation,* which refers to the written information you keep daily in order to record and monitor your progress; this includes your daily diary and your weight chart.

We talked before about the experiments conducted by Dr. Shackner, who discovered the one paramount difference between obese people and those men and women who do not suffer from overweight: namely, that thin people have something in their makeup, an instinctive or unconscious reflex, an internal mechanism that tells them after they've eaten enough, to stop eating. I call this the "enough is enough" reflex. We obese people do not have this. We are externally oriented, and when we see something tempting, we become hungry and reach out for it, even though we may have just finished eating and have no business stuffing ourselves further. We may be busting at the seams, but we still will pick up a piece of food. There is something about food in our environment that forces us to eat it. This is the one chief characteristic that identifies and separates an obese individual from someone who could never, and will never, become obese.

There are these certain engrams in the psychostructure of an obese person that compel us to eat when we shouldn't—and to alter these reflexes is the only way to solve the problem of obesity. This reflex is the result of a lifetime of conditioning, and only through a basic change in our subconscious can we learn to say "no" to food. How is this change accomplished? The overall change is achieved through my complete program of psychostructure, in which documentation is the tool we use to overcome this instinctive reaching out, and the principle is certainly not something unique; it is used in kindergarten to teach children to read and write. In brief, putting something down in a visually acceptable form helps us learn.

Of course, there is a difference between learning and remembering, and just as in kindergarten, the child who completes his homework neatly and successfully gets a star in his notebook, so also do we have *positive reinforcement* as an aid to make us instinctively, automatically, remember what we have learned.

When we fill out our daily diary, we are doing two things: first, we are developing a substitute for our lack of internal control mechanism; and, second, we are providing both positive and negative reinforcement for right and wrong behavior.

If you don't keep the diary, you will not stay on the diet. If you do keep your diary, you will stay on your diet more strictly. This was proven with an experiment using a group of obese housewives, who were told to keep track of everything they ate. Even though these women were not on a diet, they began losing weight, week after week. Why? Because for the first time in their lives, they had become aware of how much food they were eating each day. Seeing the figures before them—having to write down every morsel they consumed, realizing the extent of their overeating—all these factors brought home to each woman the grossness of her eating habits which, in turn, was responsible for the grossness of her body. Commonsense, plus a dash of feminine vanity, put the message through, and each woman began eating less each day.

The diary *is* vitally important, and together with having it with you every waking moment, you should have at home a food scale and a half-cup measure so that your portions for each meal will be accurate. You cannot trust your visual perception, because obese people look upon helpings of food as smaller than they really are. We do not view food realistically, and what would be a large portion to a thin person would seem like a very small portion to an obese eater. You must have an accurate measurement of all food at every meal so you can record your calories correctly.

None of us is perfect, and *everyone* will *always* become unstructured at some time during the program. The day you become unstructured is very important in your overall plan for weight loss.

Why is this important? First: no one can eat enough in one

episode of unstructured eating to gain what they lose in a week. You may go on an eating binge and gain ten pounds, but if you return at once to your diet, that episode will be totally wiped out in a week, often in two or three days with most people. This is true, and I have seen it happen many times with my patients.

In order to gain a pound of fat, you must eat 4000 calories. Going on a massive (I mean a really massive!) binge and consuming 16,000 calories, means you would gain four pounds. Most people would lose this four pounds the following week; so unstructured episodes are not as destructive as you might imagine, so do not become overly anxious about them.

The value of listing unstructured episodes in your diary stems from their bearing upon preventing future such episodes.

First, always write down *what* you eat, and do this while you are eating it, if at all possible. Writing it down will help diminish the amount you are eating.

Second: write down *when* you indulge in this unstructured episode. This is important to help you understand when you get into trouble. For example: four in the afternoon and nine at night are common trouble spots for most people. Many patients ask me: Can I eat an apple at 9 o'clock in the evening? The answer is *NO!* If you *do,* you only reinforce a reflex stimulation of your appetite. There's *only* one way to get rid of wanting to eat at nine in the evening: *you don't eat* at nine in the evening! Once you succumb, you will continue to be hungry at that time because you've had a positive reinforcement. If you do NOT give in to this eating urge, you will have come a long way to solving your eating problem.

Third: Write down *where* you experience your unstructured episodes. This helps you to eliminate danger spots where you find, from experience and from entries in your diary, that you inevitably indulge in an unstructured eating episode. Perhaps a certain restaurant has such a tempting lunch special, or even a constantly arousing smell inside, that you are unable to resist (freshly cooked lasagna can be devastating!)—so mark this down, and avoid this place. Concentrate only on eating establishments where you can stick to your diet menu.

Fourth: There are certain people whose chemistry reacts with our own, and we find ourselves unconsciously wanting to eat with them. Or perhaps certain people make you nervous, and you tend to overeat. By marking down in your diary with *whom* you had an unstructured episode, you'll soon see the pattern, and be able to guard yourself against a repetition.

Fifth and last: Write down how you *feel* at the time of an unstructured episode. For each of us there are characteristic feelings that cause us to overeat. This is an automatic reflex which we are not aware of, so if you record your feelings in your diary at the time of an unstructured episode, you can identify your feelings, and guard against future episodes. This is *most* important, because most patients refrain from telling their doctor how they feel, and I know from experience that many obese people suffer from depression and do not always say so. (In fact, fat people are more often than not depressed rather than jolly, as generally supposed.) So if you feel depressed and go on an eating binge (very common), write this down in your diary. If something in particular has upset you, write this down, too. Your diary is *evidence,* from which you are able to build a case against your unstructured eating episodes, and ultimately, in time, eliminate them or minimize them.

Your diary is a learning experience for you. Only through knowledge can we solve problems, and if you experience situations that cause unstructured eating episodes, only by strict documentation can you find out what they are. Whether it is one particular dish, or one restaurant, or one friend—we have a record of the experience and can eliminate that problem area from our environment. If something spells danger, you learn to be on the defensive, because, remember, we react to our environment, so it is our environment we must be careful about.

So regard your diary as your Bible: carry it everywhere, and enter everything you eat in it, from your three meals a day to any episode of unstructured eating, even if it's a handful of cashews given you by a friend. (*Very bad* indeed! eight roasted cashew nuts contain 164 calories) Always list quantities and calories and if you're at home, be sure and measure your meal portions accurately. And with unstructured episodes, remember to list the *what, when, where, who* you were with and *how* you felt at the time.

And remember that graph in the bathroom is very important. Make sure your weight chart is always in place, together with the pencil on the string, and record your weight every day. Just as you scrub your teeth, make sure you weigh yourself. After achieving your desired weight loss, use the red and yellow lines on your chart that we explained earlier. These serve as a warning to guard against any possible increase in your weight so you can correct it at once by tracing the cause and taking steps to prevent further increase.

I cannot stress too much the importance of daily exercise in losing weight. Too many people believe that diet alone can accomplish a weight loss, but believe me, often exercise alone can do that very thing, but not diet. If you were to follow my rule of two miles walking every day, and followed *only* this rule religiously, you would conquer your weight problem. If you had exercised every day of your life, you wouldn't be reading this book now because you would not be overweight. Daily exercise is the reason many of my patients are able to increase their daily calories after completing their initial desired weight loss. The increase does not result in extra weight because the additional calories are burned up by exercising. You could say the more you exercise, the less you have to restrict your calories, but this does not mean you gorge yourself on 5000 calories a day just because you walk ten miles after breakfast! There is a sensible, moderate balance between diet and exercise that should be maintained both for general health as well as weight control.

Last, *structure* is the primary theme of my program. Permanent weight control depends upon your success in adjusting your lifestyle and then adhering to the structure you set for yourself.

You do not begin a diet as if you were entering a tunnel and hoping to emerge at the other end, slender and trim. Every patient who enters my clinic is told: "Diet is not an episode of perfection, but a total change in lifestyle." Which is why psychostructure is not to be regarded as merely a diet, but as a complete rehabilitation program through which you can conquer your obesity forever.

You should not regard psychostructure as a restrictive regimen, but rather a means to assist you reorganize your life into a pattern that prevents, rather than promotes, your becoming overweight. Sure, you have limitations on what you can eat, and if you happen to indulge in an episode of unstructured eating, don't think the end of your world has happened. Merely return to your structured pattern once more. Don't feel guilty! You're only human, and until you've progressed to the point where you *automatically* control your eating habits, you will, in all probability, have occasional moments when you fall off your diet.

If this happens, merely return to your structured program at the next mealtime and continue to maintain your prescribed diet and exercise each day. This will put you back on the track again, and your momentary lapse will remain just what it is: an isolated episode instead of the beginning of an unwanted period of overeating.

Think of each week as twenty-one episodes of eating. Approach each meal, one episode at a time, and don't be concerned and castigate yourself because you overate the day before, or the week before. One meal at a time . . . one day at a time . . . one week at a time . . . one pound of weight loss at a time . . . remember!

In addition to the above three main steps (documentation, exercise, and structure), you must learn to differentiate between true hunger and appetite stimulation.

True hunger is the result of food deprivation and manifests in certain recognizable symptoms, such as fatigue. The pangs of true hunger are the body sending out signals for food, and *any* source that will provide sustenance is acceptable when you are truly hungry.

Appetite stimulation, on the other hand, is a psychological craving for certain foods, which are usually sensually appealing items like chocolate cake, ice cream, and other taste-tempting delights.

Learning to distinguish between these two impulses will be a major step forward in controlling your intake of food. Some people learn to count calories automatically to prevent reaching out for any particular item that may look tempting at first; others turn away with eyes closed and paint a mental image of themselves as they wish to be: slender and trim. Whatever means you may develop to curb your inclination for unstructured food items is fine, just as long as you arrive ultimately at a positive awareness of what you *may* and *may not* eat in order to maintain your diet and accomplish the weight loss you desire. Of immense help in this respect is your environmental restructuring, which we have dealt with earlier: the elimination of food from easy accessibility. Out of sight, out of mind . . .

Part of restructuring yourself includes eliminating from your mind all pre-conceived and common misconceptions so prevalent about weight control. I have listed these in an earlier chapter, and the facts I have given are just that: *facts*. Don't allow yourself to be influenced by misleading and erroneous claims by quacks, fly-by-night clinics, and television pitchmen whose only intention is to make a fast buck out of the tragic gullibility of the public, so many of whom happen to be overweight.

Conquering obesity is an attainable ambition if you look upon psychostructure as your future pattern of living.

Remember the three R's: *Restructuring your mind, Reprogramming your responses, and Rebuilding your body.* Think positively as you follow my program every step of the way, and twelve months from now you'll realize the indescribable elation that stems from having finally and permanently gained control over your body and achieved the slim, healthy figure you have always wanted.

Remember the Ninth Commandment of Psychostructure: *I will always remember the three R's: Restructure my mind; Reprogram my responses; and Rebuild my body.*

10. EVERY CALORIE COUNTS!

I cannot stress too highly the importance of counting calories, and if you do not already possess a book listing the calorie content of various foods, I strongly advise you to get one. An excellent calorie guide is obtainable for $1.00 from the Government Printing Office in Washington, D.C., or if you prefer, your local bookstore undoubtedly has a wide selection from which to choose.

Meanwhile, I am including a short list of commonly used food items and their respective calorie content as an aid in determining the proper portions to be used in your daily diet.

	Calories
ANCHOVIES (4 canned fillets)	28
APPLE (½ medium fresh)	35
APPLE BUTTER (1 tbsp.)	33
APPLE SAUCE (½ cup, diet pack)	50
APRICOTS (3 fresh)	55
APRICOTS (Canned diet pack, ½ cup)	56

	Calories
ARTICHOKES (½ cup cooked frozen hearts)	22
ASPARAGUS (6 spears, fresh, cooked)	20
BACON (3 slices, lean, broiled, Canadian)	50
BANANA (½ medium, 6″ long)	42
BEANS (Green, fresh cut, cooked, ½ cup)	15
BEANS (Italian, frozen, cooked, ½ cup)	23
BEEF:	
Corned (1 slice, 7″ x 1¼″ x ½″)	266
Rib roast (1 slice, 5″ x 3½″ x ¼″)	243
Rump (1 slice, 5″ x 5″ x ¼″)	235
Sirloin (1 slice, 5″ x 5″ x ¼″)	186
Steak (Club, raw, 6 oz.)	305
Flank (3 slices, 5″ x 1½″ x ¼″)	200
Round (1 slice, 3″ x 4″ x ½″)	203
Ground (Raw, 6 oz.)	271
Stew meat (Raw, chuck, boneless, 2 oz.)	210
BEEF BROTH:	
Canned, condensed, undiluted, one can	66
1 cube	6
BEEF HASH (3 oz. canned, corned)	155
BEETS (1 cup, fresh, cooked, diced)	50
BLACKBERRIES (Fresh, ½ cup)	43
BLUEBERRIES (Fresh, ½ cup)	43
BRAN FLAKES (¾ cup)	95
BROCCOLI (Frozen, chopped, cooked, ½ cup)	25
BRUSSELS SPROUTS (Frozen, cooked, 1 cup)	29
BUTTER (1 tsp.)	45
CABBAGE (Raw, shredded, 1 cup)	25
CABBAGE (Cooked, shredded, 1 cup)	35
CANTALOUPE (¼ medium)	30
CARROTS (Raw or cooked, diced, 1 cup)	45
CASABA MELON (4 oz.)	31
CATSUP (1 tbsp.)	15
CAULIFLOWER (Raw or cooked, flowerets, 1 cup)	25
CELERY (Raw, diced, 1 cup)	15
CELERY (Cooked, diced, ½ cup)	12

Calories

CHEESE:

Blue or Roquefort (1 oz.)	105
Cheddar or American (1 inch cube)	70
Cottage (½ cup)	100
Grated Parmesan (1 tbsp.)	31
Swiss (1 oz.)	105

CHERRIES (Sweet, fresh, 1 cup) ... 80

CHICKEN:

½ broiled	248
½ breast, roasted	200
1 thigh, roasted	140

CHICKEN BROTH:

Canned (14 oz.)	74
1 cube	6

CLAMS (4 large) ... 65
COD (1 piece, fresh, poached, 3″ x 3″ x 1″) ... 84
CORN FLAKES (1 cup) ... 100
CORN (1 ear, cooked) ... 70
CORN (Canned, cream style, ¼ cup) ... 45
CRAB MEAT (3 oz.) ... 89
CRANBERRY SAUCE (1 tbsp.) ... 26
CRESS (½ lb. raw, untrimmed) ... 50
CUCUMBER (1, 2″ x 7″) ... 30
DUCK (3 slices, 3½″ x 2½″ x ¼″, roasted) ... 165

EGGS:

Whole (1)	80
White only (1)	15

ENDIVE (1 cup) ... 5
FARINA (1 cup, cooked) ... 100
FLOUNDER (4 oz. frozen, poached) ... 76
FRANKFURTER (1) ... 120
FRUIT COCKTAIL (Canned, diet pack, ½ cup) ... 60
GELATIN (1 tbsp. unflavored) ... 35
GELATIN DESSERT (½ cup, low-calorie) ... 9
GRAPEFRUIT (½ medium) ... 55
GRAPEFRUIT JUICE (½ cup, fresh) ... 45

	Calories
GRAPES (1 cup, fresh)	95
HADDOCK (Fresh, broiled, 1 piece 4″ x 3″ x ½″)	100
HALIBUT (Fresh, broiled, 1 piece 4″ x 3″ x ½″)	217
HAM (Baked, 1 slice 5″ x 3″ x ½″)	53
HAM (Boiled, sliced, 1 oz.)	35
HERRING (1 oz. pickled)	60
HOMINY GRITS (1 cup, cooked)	120
HONEY (1 tbsp.)	65
HONEYDEW MELON (¼ medium)	60
KALE (1 cup, cooked)	30
KIDNEYS (Beef or lamb, 3 oz. cooked)	115
LAMB CHOP (Loin, raw, 6 oz.)	220
LEEKS (4 oz. chopped, cooked)	59
LEMON (1 medium)	20
LEMON JUICE (1 tbsp. fresh)	5
LIVER:	
Cooked beef (4 oz.)	260
Cooked chicken (4 oz.)	146
Cooked pork (4 oz.)	273
LOBSTER (½ cup, canned)	80
MANDARIN ORANGES (¼ cup, diet pack)	25
MARGARINE (1 tbsp.)	100
MIXED VEGETABLES (Frozen, cooked, ½ cup)	55
MUSHROOMS (6 large, fresh)	14
OAT CEREAL (1 cup, cooked)	100
OLIVES (Green or ripe, 3 medium)	10
ONION (1 medium)	40
ONION (Green, 6 small)	20
ORANGE (1 medium)	70
ORANGE JUICE (½ cup, fresh)	55
OYSTERS (14-18, raw, medium)	160
PAPAYA (1 cup, fresh, cubed)	70
PARSLEY (1 tbsp. fresh, chopped)	1
PARSNIPS (½ cup, cooked, diced)	50
PEACHES (1 whole, fresh, medium)	35
PEACHES (Diet pack, 2 halves, and 2 tbsp. syrup)	54

Calories

PEANUT BUTTER (1 tbsp.)	95
PEARS (½, fresh, medium)	50
PEARS (Canned, diet pack, 2 halves, 2 tbsp. syrup)	62
PEAS (Fresh, green, cooked, ½ cup)	55
PEPPERS (Sweet, raw, green, 1 medium)	15
PICKLES (1 dill, 5″)	15
PICKLES (1 sweet, 3″)	30
PINEAPPLE (Fresh, diced, 1 cup)	75
PINEAPPLE (Canned diet pack, ¼ cup)	57
PLUMS (1 whole, fresh, medium)	25
PLUMS (Canned diet pack, 3 plums, 2 tbsp. syrup)	75
POTATOES:	
Baked, without skin (1 medium)	90
Boiled, peeled, 1 medium	105
Mashed with milk only (½ cup)	70
PRUNES (4 uncooked)	70
PUMPKIN (1 cup, canned)	75
RADISHES (4 small)	5
RASPBERRIES (1 cup, red, fresh)	70
RICE:	
1 cup white, cooked	185
⅔ cup, brown, cooked	100
Wild, cooked, ½ cup	73
RICE CEREAL, PUFFED (1 cup)	55
RUTABAGAS (½ cup, cooked, cubed)	25
SALAD DRESSING:	
Low calorie Blue cheese (1 tbsp.)	15
Low calorie French (1 tbsp.)	9
Low calorie Thousand Island (1 tbsp.)	33
SALMON (½ cup, canned)	120
SARDINES (4, canned)	100
SAUERKRAUT (1 cup, canned)	32
SCALLOPS (6 medium fresh)	105
SHREDDED WHEAT (1 biscuit)	90
SHRIMPS (7 medium size, fresh)	100
SOLE (4 oz. frozen, poached)	88

	Calories
SPINACH (1 cup, cooked, fresh)	40
SQUASH (1 cup, cooked)	30
STRAWBERRIES (1 cup, fresh)	55
SUCCOTASH (½ cup cooked)	87
SWEET POTATOES (½ boiled, medium)	85
TANGERINE (1 large)	40
TOMATOES (1 fresh, medium)	35
TUNA (½ cup, drained, canned in water)	109
TURNIPS (1 cup, white, cooked)	35
TURKEY (Roast breast, 1 slice 4″ x 3″ x ¼″)	134
VEAL (Chop, loin, raw, 6 oz.)	180
WATERMELON (1 wedge 4″ x 4″ x 8″)	115
WHEAT CEREAL, PUFFED (1 cup)	55
YAMS (4 oz. raw, peeled)	115
YOGURT (1 cup diet)	120

ALCOHOLIC BEVERAGES

	Calories
ALE, mild, 8 oz.	98
BEER, 8 oz.	114
WINES:	
Champagne, brut, 3 oz.	75
Champagne, extra dry, 3 oz.	87
Dubonnet, 3 oz.	96
Dry Marsala, 3 oz.	162
Sweet Marsala, 3 oz.	182
Muscatel, 4 oz.	158
Port, 4 oz.	158
Red wine, dry, 3 oz.	69
Sake, 3 oz.	75
Sherry, domestic, 3½ oz.	84
Dry vermouth, 3½ oz.	105
Sweet vermouth, 3½ oz.	167
White wine, dry, 3 oz.	74

Calories

LIQUEURS AND CORDIALS (BOLS):
Creme de Cacao, 1 oz.   101
Creme de Menthe, 1 oz.   112
Curaçao, 1 oz.   100
Drambuie, 1 oz.   110
Tia Maria, 1 oz.   113

SPIRITS:
Bourbon, brandy, Cognac, Canadian whiskey, gin, rye,
rum, Scotch, tequila and vodka are all carbohydrate free!
The calories they contain depend upon the proof.
80 proof, 1 oz.   67
84 proof, 1 oz.   70
90 proof, 1 oz.   75
94 proof, 1 oz.   78
97 proof, 1 oz.   81
100 proof, 1 oz.   83

Remember the Tenth Commandment of Psychostructure:
I will always remember that every calorie counts!

INDEX